# Decision Sciences in Bioinformatics

Bioinformatics deals with computational and mathematical approaches for understanding and processing biological data. This book highlights the computational procedures and the applications evolving around biological data, including usage of decision sciences for a variety of applications, namely text mining, "OMIC" sciences, systems biology, analyzing biological/medical images, computer-aided diagnosis/ treatment of diseases, decision sciences for public health with COVID-19 data, bio-diversity, smart wearables, personalized medicine, data deluge issues, and knowledge management.

Key Features:

- Presents exclusive material on decision sciences in bioinformatics
- Highlights the computational procedures and applications evolving around biological data
- Provides solutions to problems in bioinformatics with decision sciences
- Addresses the research gaps in bioinformatics
- Includes case studies emphasizing societal needs

This book is aimed at researchers and graduate students in bioinformatics and data analytics.

# Decision Sciences in Bioinformatics

## Theory and Practice

Edited by S. Sumathi, Suresh V. Rajappa,
B. Vinoth Kumar, Surekha P., and P. Sivakumar

CRC Press
Taylor & Francis Group
Boca Raton London New York

CRC Press is an imprint of the
Taylor & Francis Group, an **informa** business

Designed cover image: Shutterstock

First edition published 2026
by CRC Press
2385 NW Executive Center Drive, Suite 320, Boca Raton FL 33431

and by CRC Press
4 Park Square, Milton Park, Abingdon, Oxon, OX14 4RN

*CRC Press is an imprint of Taylor & Francis Group, LLC*



ISBN: 9781032535494 (hbk)
ISBN: 9781032582160 (pbk)
ISBN: 9781003449058 (ebk)

DOI: 10.1201/9781003449058

Typeset in Times
by Newgen Publishing UK

# Contents

# Preface

Bioinformatics, at the intersection of computational and mathematical disciplines, plays a pivotal role in decoding biological data. This synergy is essential for sustaining and advancing biological processes that support life on Earth. With the exponential growth of biological data, there is a pressing need for sophisticated computational methods to store, manage, and analyze this information. This book explores these computational techniques and their practical applications, providing an in-depth look at how bioinformatics and decision sciences can tackle a range of challenges. The aim is to equip researchers, practitioners, and students with the necessary tools and knowledge to navigate and contribute to this dynamic field.

Chapter 1 introduces a Semantic Data Fabric (SDF) framework that utilizes AI and ontologies for the automated integration of healthcare data. This cutting-edge approach improves risk prognosis, enables personalized preventive care, and simplifies data interpretation for healthcare professionals. By aligning global medical standards with machine learning algorithms, the SDF framework has the potential to transform healthcare decision-making, enhance patient outcomes, and ensure data privacy and compliance. The chapter delves into the technical aspects of the SDF framework, its implementation, and case studies that highlight its effectiveness in real-world healthcare settings.

Chapter 2 describes an innovative method for designing 2.45 GHz fractal antennas used in implantable and wearable COVID-19 health monitoring devices. The gasket-shaped array, modeled using MATLAB software, achieves a reflection coefficient of up to -35 dB at 2.45 GHz, effectively mitigating losses caused by human body interaction. This chapter provides a detailed overview of the design process, the challenges faced, and the solutions developed to optimize antenna performance. It also discusses the potential applications of these antennas in continuous health monitoring and early disease detection, contributing to improved patient care and health outcomes.

Chapter 3 focuses on a hybrid model combining Convolutional Neural Networks (CNN) and Long Short-Term Memory (LSTM) networks for thyroid prediction. The CNN extracts spatial features from clinical data, while the LSTM captures temporal patterns, integrating both methods to enhance prediction accuracy. This chapter explains the underlying principles of CNN and LSTM, their integration into a cohesive model, and the advantages of this hybrid approach. It includes experimental results, comparative analyses, and discussions on how this model can be applied to other medical prediction scenarios, offering insights into its broader applicability.

Chapter 4 presents a hybrid Generative Adversarial Network (GAN) model that integrates Long Short-Term Memory (LSTM) and Residual Network (ResNet) for COVID-19 classification in CT images. This model improves detection accuracy and robustness, with LSTM capturing spatial features and ResNet providing precise discrimination, as evidenced by experimental results. The chapter provides a comprehensive guide to the GAN architecture, the integration process of LSTM and ResNet, and the experimental setup. It also highlights the potential of this model to be adapted for other medical imaging applications, demonstrating its versatility and impact on diagnostic accuracy.

Chapter 5 proposes a novel disease diagnosis approach using a dynamic weighted ensemble with Teaching-Learning-Based Optimization (TLBO). By combining Logistic Regression, K-Nearest Neighbors, Decision Tree, and Support Vector Machine models, the TLBO algorithm updates ensemble composition and weights, boosting accuracy and adaptability. Evaluations across various datasets confirm its effectiveness. This chapter covers the theoretical foundation of TLBO, the process of creating dynamic weighted ensembles, and the application of this method to different disease datasets. It also includes practical examples and case studies, providing a thorough understanding of how this approach can be implemented and its potential benefits in disease diagnosis.

Chapter 6 discusses the use of neuroimaging biomarkers for diagnosing Alzheimer's disease (AD) and reviews various machine learning algorithms employed for this purpose. It also explores future research directions, including personalized medicine and multimodal imaging applications. This chapter provides an in-depth look at the different types of neuroimaging techniques, the biomarkers used for AD diagnosis, and the machine learning models that have shown promise in this area. It also examines the challenges and opportunities in advancing AD research, offering a roadmap for future studies and innovations in neuroimaging and machine learning.

Chapter 7 addresses the detection of fake news in healthcare, using the COVID-19 pandemic as a case study, and outlines mitigation techniques to manage misinformation. This chapter discusses the impact of fake news on public health, the challenges in detecting and combating misinformation, and the development of algorithms to identify fake news. It also explores strategies for public education and awareness, highlighting the importance of accurate information dissemination in healthcare. The chapter provides insights into the intersection of data science and communication, emphasizing the role of technology in ensuring the integrity of healthcare information.

Chapter 8 tackles the challenges of data deluge in medical care IoT devices and big data in healthcare. It discusses modern techniques like machine learning and artificial intelligence to overcome these issues and proposes systematic approaches to improve the triaging of transmissions to reduce data overload. This chapter covers the technical aspects of managing large-scale data, the integration of IoT devices in healthcare, and the implementation of AI-driven solutions to streamline data processing. It also includes case studies and practical examples, demonstrating the effectiveness of these techniques in real-world scenarios and their potential to transform healthcare data management.

Chapter 9 explores the application of deep learning in identifying plant species and detecting diseases, which is crucial for preventing losses and enhancing agricultural quality and yield. The proposed system uses the GoogleNet model, providing an efficient alternative to manual inspections, and highlights research gaps and advancements in early plant disease detection. This chapter discusses the significance of plant health monitoring, the challenges in early disease detection, and the development of deep learning models for this purpose. It also presents experimental results, comparative analyses, and future research directions, emphasizing the impact of technology on agriculture and food security.

This book underscores the main applications of bioinformatics and decision sciences, from healthcare data integration and health monitoring device design to thyroid prediction, COVID-19 classification, disease diagnosis, fake news detection, neuroimaging for Alzheimer's, managing data deluge in medical IoT devices, and plant species identification and disease detection. These diverse yet interconnected topics make this book an invaluable resource for data scientists, industry practitioners, bioinformatics statisticians, medical informaticists, research scholars, and graduate students. By presenting these varied applications, we aim to inspire further research and innovation in harnessing AI and decision sciences to address real-world challenges, ultimately advancing the field of bioinformatics and improving life on our planet. The book seeks to provide readers with comprehensive knowledge and practical insights, fostering a deeper understanding of the role of bioinformatics and decision sciences in today's data-driven world.

# About the Editors

**S. Sumathi** is a Professor in the Department of Electrical and Electronics Engineering, PSG College of Technology, Coimbatore with 34 years of teaching and research experience. Her research interests include Neural Networks, Fuzzy Systems and Genetic Algorithms, Pattern Recognition and Classification, Data Warehousing and Data Mining, Operating systems, and Parallel Computing. She is the author of more than 40 papers in refereed journals and international conferences. She has authored 10 books with reputed publishers such as Springer, CRC Press, and Nova Publishers.

**Suresh V. Rajappa** PhD PMP MBA is a seasoned senior IT management consulting professional with 25 years' experience leading large global IT programs and projects in IT Strategy, Finance IT (FINTECH) Transformation Strategy, BI and data warehousing/Data Analytics and Management for multiple fortune 100 clients across diverse industries, generating millions of dollars to top and bottom lines. Dr. Suresh Rajappa has been successful at recruiting and leading onshore/offshore cross-cultural teams to deliver complex enterprise-wide solutions within tight deadlines and budgets. He is highly effective at breaking down strategic program/project initiatives into tactical plans and processes to achieve aggressive customer goals. He excels at leveraging strategic partnerships, global resources, process improvements, and best practices to maximize project delivery performance and ROI. He is an inspirational, solution-focused leader with exceptional ability managing multimillion-dollar P&Ls/budgets and change management initiatives. As an adjunct professor, Dr. Suresh Rajappa teaches data science for graduate and doctoral students at PSG College of Technology. His Industry specializations include Utility, Finance (Banking and Insurance), and HiTech Manufacturing. He is a frequent speaker at Microsoft PASS conferences, SAP Financials, and SAP TechEd conferences on Data Analytics related topics. He also teaches Data Analytics and IT Project Management to undergraduate and graduate level students. He has also been a keynote speaker at an International Conference on Artificial Intelligence, Smart Grid, and Smart City Applications.

**B. Vinoth Kumar** is a Professor in the Department of Information Technology at PSG College of Technology, with 20 years of experience. His current research interests include Computational Intelligence, Memetic Algorithms, Affective Computing, and Image Processing. He has authored over 60 papers in refereed journals and international conferences. Additionally, he has edited eight books published by reputed publishers such as Springer and CRC Press. He also serves as a guest editor and reviewer for numerous journals from leading publishers including IEEE, Elsevier, Springer, Inderscience, and De Gruyter.

**Surekha P.** is an Assistant Professor (Sr. Gr) in the Department of Electrical and Electronics Engineering, Amrita School of Engineering, Bengaluru, Amrita Vishwa Vidyapeetham, India with 20 years of experience in teaching, industry, and research. She has published 35 papers in International and National journals and conferences.

She has authored seven books with leading publishers such as CRC Press and Springer. Her research interests include Control Systems, Computational Intelligence, Machine Learning, Signal and Image Processing, Embedded Systems, Real-time operating systems, and Virtual Instrumentation.

**P. Sivakumar** is an Assistant Professor (Sl.Gr) in the Department of Electrical and Electronics Engineering, PSG College of Technology, Coimbatore with 18 years of teaching and research experience. He completed his PhD in Electrical Engineering with a specialization in Automotive Embedded Software in the year 2018 from Anna University, PSG College of Technology. His research interests include Embedded Systems, Model-based Design, and Model-based Testing of Automotive Software, Automotive Software Development, Fog and Edge Computing. He serves as a Guest Editor/Reviewer of journals with leading publishers such as Inderscience.

# Contributors

**Anuradha J.**, School of Computer Science and Engineering, Vellore Institute of Technology, Vellore, India.

**Bhuvaneswari Velumani**, Department of Computer Applications, Bharathiar University, India

**Chandrasekaran K.**, National Institute of Technology Karnataka, Surathkal, India

**Eswaran Sivaraman**, Department of Electrical and Computer Engineering, Curtin University Malaysia, Miri, Sarawak, Malaysia

**Jayachandran Uma Maheswari**, School of Computer Science and Engineering, Vellore Institute of Technology, Chennai, Tamil Nadu, India

**Karthikeyan Thiyagarajan**, Assistant Professor, Department of Information Technology, University of Technology and Applied Sciences, Salalah, Oman

**Krishnamoorthy Somasundaram**, School of Computer Science and Engineering, Vellore Institute of Technology, Vellore, India

**Lissa Mahimadass**, Department of Computer Applications, Bharathiar University, Coimbatore, India

**Malliga L.**, Malla Reddy Engineering College for Women, Hyderabad, India

**Mathiyalagan P.**, Sri Ramakrishna, Engineering College, Coimbatore, India

**Ms. S. Biruntha**, Sri Krishna College of Engineering and Technology, Coimbatore, India

**Murugan Murali**, Director of Engineering, Macy's, Georgia-30005, USA.

**Nalini N.**, School of Computer Science and Engineering, Vellore Institute of Technology, Vellore, India.

**Palanisamy Prema**, Velalar College of Engineering and Technology, Erode, India

**Paulraj Sivakumar**, School of Computer Science and Engineering, Vellore Institute of Technology, Chennai, India

**Periyasamy Baskaran**, School of Computer Science and Engineering, Vellore Institute of Technology, Vellore, India

**Rajalakshmi S**, Dr. NGP Institute of Technology, Coimbatore, India

**Rajarajeshwari K.C.**, Dr Mahalingam College of Engineering and Technology, Pollachi, India.

**Rama Abirami, K.**, Curtin University, Lecturer, Department of Electrical and Computer Engineering, Malaysia

**Ramalingaswamy Cheruku**, Department of Computer Science and Engineering, National Institute of Technology, Warangal, India

**Ramamoorthy Arun Kumar**, Digital Forensics & Cyber Security, University of South Wales, Treforest, United Kingdom

**Sadhanaa Balaji**, Aarupadai Veedu Medical College and Hospital, Pondicherry, India.

**Saravanakumar N.**, Dr Mahalingam College of Engineering and Technology, Pollachi, India

**Selvaraj Nagendra Prabhu**, Department of Computational Intelligence, School of Computing, SRM Institute of Science and Technology, Kattankulathur, Chennai, India

**Shivashankar G. (third)** Department of Computational Intelligence, SRM Institute of Science and Technology, Chennai, India

**Sivaramakrishnan Sangameswaran**, Amazon Inc, VA, USA

**Srihari Govindarajan**, Chief executive Officer, Kloud Logic Inc, CA, USA

**Srinivas Arukonda**, Assistant Professor SRM University-AP, Andhra Pradesh, India

**Sriram Sridevi**, School of Computer Science and Engineering, Vellore Institute of Technology, Vellore, India

**Usha Divakarla**, NMAM Institute of Technology, Nitte, Karkala, India

**Venkatesh B.**, Department of Computer Science and Engineering, BVRIT Hyderabad College of Engineering for Women, Hyderabad, India

**Vijeyakumar K.N.**, Dr Mahalingam College of Engineering and Technology, Pollachi, India

# 1 Semantic Data Fabric for Automated Health Care Data Integration Using AI for Risk Prognosis and Preventive Care

*M. Lissa and V. Bhuvaneswari*

## 1.1 INTRODUCTION

The healthcare industry has been facing challenges in integrating vast amounts of diverse data from various sources [1, 2]. Semantic Data Fabric (SDF) is a promising solution to this problem that uses artificial intelligence (AI) algorithms to automatically integrate and interpret complex healthcare data [3]. This technology can facilitate risk prognosis and preventive care. This chapter focuses on developing a Semantic Data Fabric for Automated Health Care Data Integration using AI for Risk Prognosis and Preventive Care, specifically targeting the challenges of prognosis tracking and adverse effect monitoring in cancer diseases.

Prognosis tracking and adverse effect monitoring play critical roles in cancer disease management, providing valuable insights for healthcare professionals to make informed decisions and optimize patient care [4]. Accurately tracking the prognosis and monitoring adverse effects are vital for tailoring treatment plans and ensuring positive patient outcomes. However, these tasks are often complicated due to the diverse characteristics of cancer diseases and the multitude of data sources involved.

The objectives of this chapter are threefold [1]. First, to explore the background and significance of prognosis tracking and adverse effect monitoring in cancer diseases. By highlighting the importance of these aspects in guiding treatment decisions and improving patient outcomes, we lay the foundation for the development of an integrated tool that addresses these challenges.

Second, to focus on the development of a comprehensive Semantic Data Fabric that integrates ontology modeling and AI algorithms [3]. The Semantic Data Fabric serves as a framework for automated health care data integration and analysis, facilitating risk prognosis and preventive care. By leveraging ontologies, which provide standardized terminologies and structured representations of domain-specific

DOI: 10.1201/9781003449058-1

knowledge, we achieve a unified view of patient data, enabling seamless integration and analysis.

Lastly, the structure of the chapter is outlined to provide a roadmap for the subsequent sections [5]. The chapter encompasses various aspects of the tool's development, including methodology, implementation details, and case studies. This helps to explore how the Semantic Data Fabric with ontology integration enhances prognosis tracking, enables adverse effect monitoring, and supports clinical decision-making.

By the end of this chapter, it will have enabled a comprehensive understanding of the significance of prognosis tracking and adverse effect monitoring in cancer diseases [6]. It will also show insights into the development and integration of ontologies within the Semantic Data Fabric, and how this integration enhances the overall cancer disease management process.

Through the integration of prognosis tracking, adverse effect monitoring, and ontology integration within the Semantic Data Fabric, this chapter presents a novel approach to automated health care data integration using AI [7]. The proposed solution has the potential to revolutionize cancer disease management, improve treatment outcomes, and provide healthcare professionals with valuable insights for personalized patient care.

## 1.2 BACKGROUND AND CHALLENGES IN CANCER DISEASE MANAGEMENT

Cancer disease management presents unique challenges for physicians, requiring them to navigate complex data sources and make informed decisions for personalized treatment planning and monitoring [8]. These challenges arise from the intricate nature of cancer diseases, the diversity of patient data, and the need for comprehensive assessments of disease severities, adverse effects, and comorbidity conditions.

### 1.2.1 Prognosis Tracking and Adverse Effect Monitoring Challenges

In the realm of cancer disease management, physicians encounter various challenges when it comes to prognosis tracking and adverse effect monitoring [9]. Prognosis tracking involves assessing the severity and progression of the disease, predicting treatment outcomes, and understanding the potential risks faced by patients. Adverse effect monitoring, on the other hand, focuses on identifying and managing the unintended consequences of treatments, medications, or the disease itself.

The challenges physicians face in these areas are multifaceted [10]. Accessing and integrating diverse data sources, such as clinical parameters, imaging data, genetic profiles, and treatment records, can be time-consuming and complex. Traditional relational databases often pose difficulties in retrieving comprehensive diagnostic summaries and assessing disease severities due to their relational nature and complex data structures. Similarly, identifying and linking adverse effects to specific treatments or comorbidity conditions can be challenging, as relevant information is scattered across various database tables and lacks standardized terminology.

### 1.2.2 Importance of Personalized Treatment Planning and Monitoring for Improved Patient Outcomes

Personalized treatment planning and monitoring are critical components of cancer disease management [11]. Tailoring treatment plans to individual patients can lead to improved outcomes and patient satisfaction. However, achieving this level of personalization requires comprehensive and accurate assessment of disease severities, identification of adverse effects, and consideration of comorbidity conditions.

By understanding the challenges and addressing them effectively, physicians can enhance their ability to provide personalized treatment plans that consider the specific needs and characteristics of each patient [12]. Accurate prognosis tracking and adverse effect monitoring contribute to treatment optimization, allowing healthcare professionals to make well-informed decisions that maximize efficacy while minimizing potential risks.

### 1.2.3 IoT-Relevant Healthcare Data and Data Integration Challenges

The rise of the Internet of Things (IoT) has brought about significant advancements in healthcare, generating vast amounts of data from various sources such as wearable devices, remote monitoring systems, and sensor-equipped medical devices [13]. This IoT-relevant healthcare data holds immense potential for improving patient care, enabling early detection of diseases, and facilitating real-time monitoring of health conditions. However, integrating this diverse and voluminous data into existing healthcare systems poses considerable challenges.

One major challenge is data interoperability, as IoT devices and systems often employ different communication protocols and data formats [14]. The lack of standardization and compatibility hampers the seamless integration of IoT-generated data into the healthcare ecosystem. Healthcare professionals must grapple with the task of harmonizing and integrating data from different IoT devices to obtain a comprehensive view of the patient's health status.

In particular, image data plays a vital role in diagnosing and monitoring various diseases [15]. However, integrating image data into healthcare systems presents additional challenges. Medical images are typically large, complex, and require specialized software for analysis. Furthermore, the integration of image data with other patient information, such as electronic health records and laboratory results, can be arduous due to the need for efficient storage, transmission, and retrieval of these data types.

Addressing these challenges requires innovative approaches to data integration [16]. Standardization efforts, such as the use of common data models and interoperability standards, can facilitate the seamless exchange and integration of IoT-relevant healthcare data. Additionally, advanced technologies such as artificial intelligence and machine learning can aid in automating the integration process, extracting meaningful insights from diverse datasets, and supporting clinical decision-making.

By overcoming the challenges related to data interoperability and image data integration, healthcare professionals can unlock the full potential of IoT-relevant data in improving patient care, early disease detection, and personalized treatment strategies [17].

### 1.2.4 Overview of the Need for Integrated Tools that Leverage Ontologies

To overcome the challenges faced by physicians in prognosis tracking, adverse effect monitoring, and personalized treatment planning, the integration of tools that leverage ontologies is crucial [18]. Ontologies provide a structured representation of medical knowledge, standardized terminologies, and semantic relationships [19]. Integrating ontologies with data sources allows for a more intuitive and efficient retrieval and analysis process.

Semantic technologies, such as ontologies, enable the integration of disparate data sources by harmonizing and standardizing terminology [20]. They facilitate the linking of diagnostic summaries, disease severities, adverse effects, and comorbidity conditions with patient-specific characteristics, treatments, and outcomes. By leveraging semantic technologies, physicians gain access to a unified and holistic view of patient data, enabling more efficient decision-making, personalized treatment planning, and monitoring of adverse effects.

However, by leveraging semantic technologies and integrating tools that utilize ontologies, physicians can overcome these challenges [21]. The use of ontologies facilitates the integration and standardization of diverse data sources, improving data retrieval and analysis. The next section explores how semantic technologies can be helpful in addressing these challenges and enhancing cancer disease management practices.

## 1.3 PROTOTYPE ARCHITECTURE DEVELOPMENT AND FUNCTIONALITY

The prototype architecture for prognosis tracking and adverse effect monitoring is designed to address the challenges faced by physicians in cancer disease management [22]. It consists of several key components and layers that work together to provide a comprehensive solution as shown in Figure 1.1.

The developed prototype serves as an innovative tool to streamline prognosis tracking and adverse effect monitoring in cancer diseases [23]. It includes the following components:

a. **Overview of the Developed Prototype for Prognosis Tracking and Adverse Effect Monitoring**

   **User Interface:** The user interface provides healthcare professionals with a user-friendly platform to interact with the prototype [24]. It allows them to input patient data, view analysis results, and access personalized treatment recommendations.

   **Data Collection:** The prototype allows healthcare professionals to input various parameters such as vital signs, laboratory results, imaging reports,

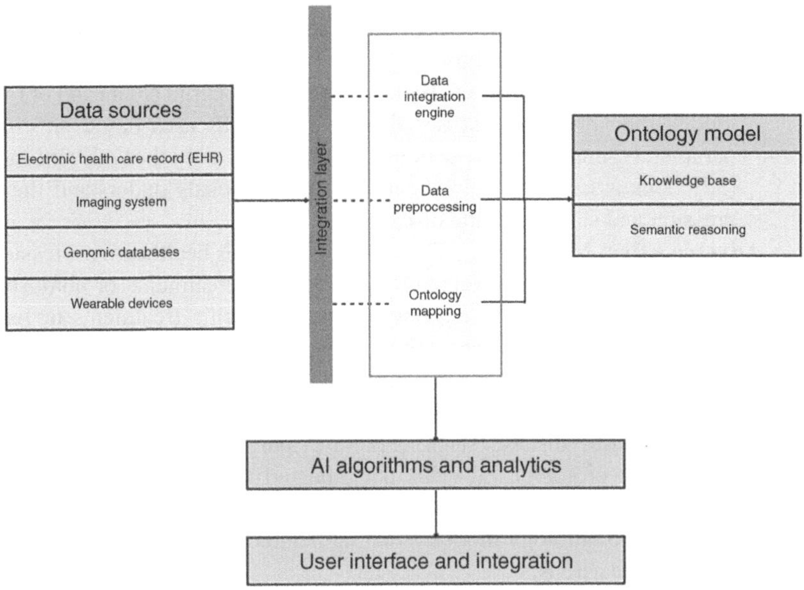


**FIGURE 1.1** Overview of Semantic Data Fabric prototype architecture.

genomic information, and treatment history [25]. These input parameters capture essential aspects of the patient's health status

**Data Analysis:** The prototype employs advanced data analysis techniques, including machine learning algorithms and statistical analysis, to derive meaningful insights from the collected patient data [26]. These techniques help identify patterns, correlations, and potential risk factors related to disease severity and adverse effects.

**Visualization:** The prototype provides visualization capabilities to present the analyzed data and insights in a user-friendly manner [27]. It includes interactive charts, graphs, and reports that enable healthcare professionals to interpret and communicate the findings effectively.

**Prototype Functionalities**

The prototype encompasses a range of functionalities to support prognosis tracking and adverse effect monitoring:

**Data Integration:** The prototype integrates and harmonizes data from various sources, such as electronic health records, imaging systems, genomic databases, and wearable devices [28]. This integration ensures a comprehensive view of the patient's health information.

**Ontology Integration:** The prototype incorporates an ontology model that provides a structured representation of medical knowledge, disease classifications, treatment guidelines, adverse effect profiles, and standardized terminologies [29–31]. This integration enables standardized data representation and supports accurate disease severity assessment and treatment recommendations.

**Disease Severity Assessment:** By leveraging the integrated data and ontology model, the prototype assesses the severity of diseases based on clinical parameters, imaging data, genomic information, and other relevant factors [32]. This assessment helps healthcare professionals understand the progression and severity of the disease.

**Adverse Effect Monitoring:** The prototype enables healthcare professionals to monitor and track adverse effects related to treatments or comorbidity conditions [33]. It links adverse effects to specific treatments or patient characteristics, facilitating proactive management and personalized treatment adjustments.

**Personalized Treatment Recommendations:** Based on the patient's unique characteristics, disease stage, genomic markers, and potential adverse effects, the prototype provides personalized treatment recommendations [34]. These recommendations are derived from evidence-based guidelines stored in the ontology model, assisting healthcare professionals in making informed decisions.

**b. Prototype Integrates an Ontology Model**

The prototype integrates an ontology model to enhance disease severity assessment and treatment solutions [35]. The ontology model serves as a knowledge repository and provides a structured representation of medical knowledge, disease classifications, treatment guidelines, adverse effect profiles, and standardized terminologies [36].

By aligning patient data with the ontology's knowledge base, the prototype establishes semantic relationships and utilizes standardized terminologies, improving the accuracy and consistency of data analysis [37]. This integration allows the prototype to categorize and analyze patient data based on a standardized framework, facilitating more precise disease severity assessment and personalized treatment recommendations.

The ontology model enhances the prototype's ability to access comprehensive information about diseases, treatments, and potential adverse effects [38]. It provides a foundation for evidence-based decision-making and supports healthcare professionals in making informed treatment plans.

**c. Semantic Data Fabric and AI: An Overview**

Semantic Data Fabric is a technology framework that combines the power of semantics, data integration, and analytics to enable efficient and meaningful integration of heterogeneous healthcare data. SDF utilizes ontologies, which are structured representations of knowledge, to provide a common understanding and standardization of data elements and their relationships. By leveraging ontologies, SDF allows for the integration and interpretation of diverse healthcare data from various sources [39].

In the context of the developed prototype, SDF plays a crucial role in facilitating the integration and harmonization of data from electronic health records, imaging systems, genomic databases, and wearable devices. The use of ontologies enables standardized data representation and semantic querying, leading to more accurate disease severity assessment and personalized treatment recommendations.

d. **Artificial Intelligence (AI)**
   Artificial intelligence, particularly machine learning algorithms and statistical analysis, plays a vital role in the prototype architecture. AI algorithms enable the analysis of large volumes of patient data, identify patterns, correlations, and potential risk factors, and generate insights for prognosis tracking and adverse effect monitoring.

Machine learning algorithms are employed to develop predictive models that can assess disease severity and predict treatment outcomes based on patient characteristics and input parameters. Statistical analysis techniques are utilized to derive meaningful insights from aggregated patient data and identify trends or associations between clinical parameters and adverse effects.

The integration of AI within the prototype enhances decision-making by providing healthcare professionals with evidence-based recommendations for personalized treatment plans. AI algorithms also assist in risk assessment, enabling proactive monitoring and interventions to mitigate potential adverse effects.

By combining the capabilities of SDF and AI, the prototype architecture leverages semantic integration, standardized data representation, and advanced analytics to support prognosis tracking and adverse effect monitoring in cancer disease management.

## 1.4 SEMANTIC DATA FABRIC FOR HEALTHCARE DATA INTEGRATION

The integration of diverse healthcare data poses significant challenges due to the heterogeneity and complexity of the information. Semantic Data Fabric (SDF) emerges as a powerful solution to address these challenges by leveraging semantic relationships and advanced reasoning capabilities. In the context of healthcare data integration, SDF offers a unified and holistic approach to integrating, interpreting, and analyzing healthcare data. This section focuses on the application of Semantic Data Fabric for Healthcare Data Integration and explores its benefits in risk prognosis and preventive care.

a. **Benefits of Semantic Data Fabric for Healthcare Data Integration:**
   i. **Flexibility and Extensibility:**
      Semantic Data Fabric allows for flexible and extensible data integration by capturing the semantic relationships between entities. It enables the addition of new concepts, attributes, and relationships without disrupting the existing data structure, providing adaptability to evolving healthcare domains.

ii. **Semantic Relationships:**
The inclusion of semantic relationships in the data integration process goes beyond simple structural relationships. Semantic Data Fabric captures deeper insights into how entities are related, enabling more intelligent querying, reasoning, and inference. This semantic understanding enhances decision-making, knowledge discovery, and predictive analysis.

iii. **Interoperability and Integration:**
Semantic Data Fabric facilitates interoperability by establishing a common vocabulary and standardized semantics. It enables the integration of diverse healthcare data sources by mapping their concepts and relationships to a shared ontology. This interoperability enhances data exchange, knowledge sharing, and collaboration across different systems and organizations.

iv. **Advanced Reasoning and Inference:**
Semantic Data Fabric supports advanced reasoning capabilities, such as deduction, classification, and inference. By capturing explicit semantic relationships, it enables the system to derive new knowledge from existing data. This reasoning capability enhances decision-making, identifies patterns, correlations, and hidden insights, and supports predictive analysis in healthcare applications.

v. **Enhanced Data Analysis and Insights:**
Semantic Data Fabric enriches data analysis by providing a semantic layer that enhances the accuracy and relevance of results. By incorporating domain knowledge and context, it improves the interpretation and understanding of data. Semantic relationships help in identifying meaningful patterns, correlations, and insights that may not be apparent in the raw data alone.

vi. **Conceptual Clarity and Standardized Semantics**
Semantic Data Fabric ensures conceptual clarity by providing explicit definitions, constraints, and hierarchies. It establishes a shared understanding of concepts, attributes, and relationships within a specific healthcare domain. This clarity promotes effective communication, consistency in data representation, and accurate data interpretation.

## 1.5 ONTOLOGY INTEGRATION FOR CANCER DISEASES

Ontology provides a solution-oriented approach compared to a traditional relational database system. While relational databases excel at structuring and organizing data, they often fall short in capturing the rich semantic relationships and knowledge that exist within complex domains like healthcare as shown in Figure 1.2. Ontologies, on the other hand, offer a more flexible and expressive framework for representing and reasoning about data. By capturing explicit relationships and semantics, ontologies enable a deeper understanding of the data, facilitating advanced reasoning, integration, and interoperability. They allow for the representation of domain-specific knowledge, hierarchies, and constraints, providing a standardized and shared

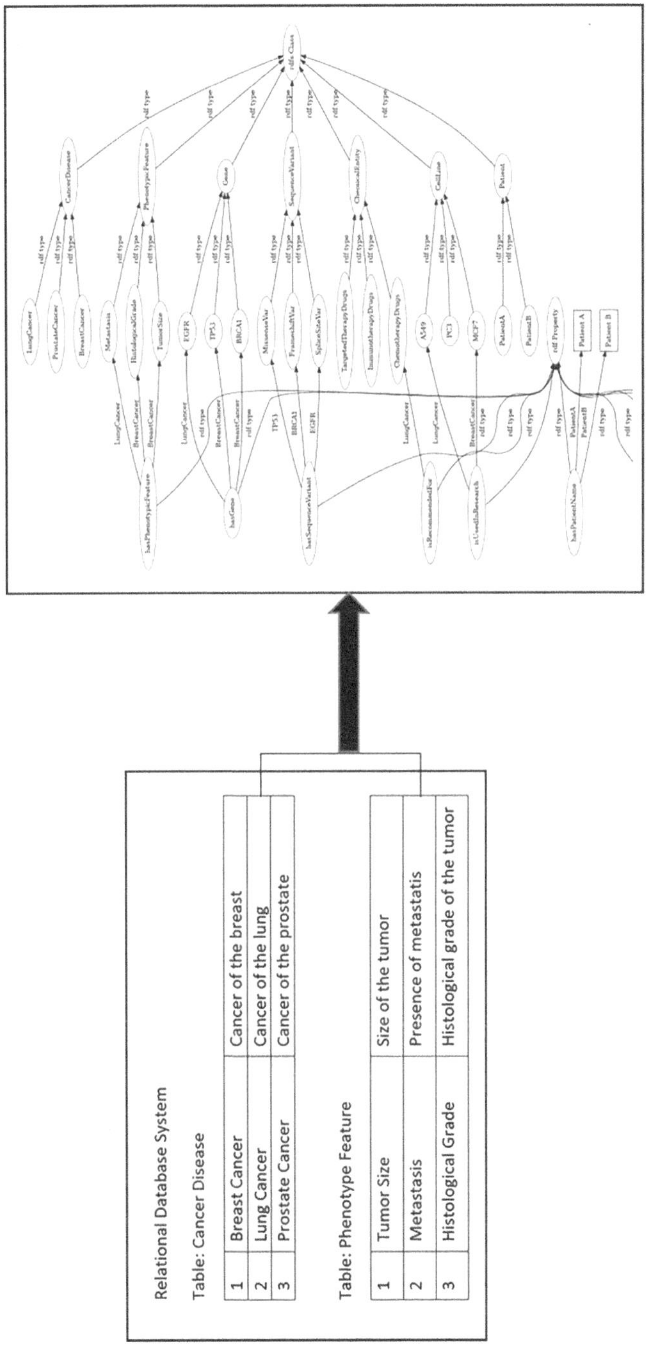


**FIGURE 1.2** Knowledge model over traditional approach.

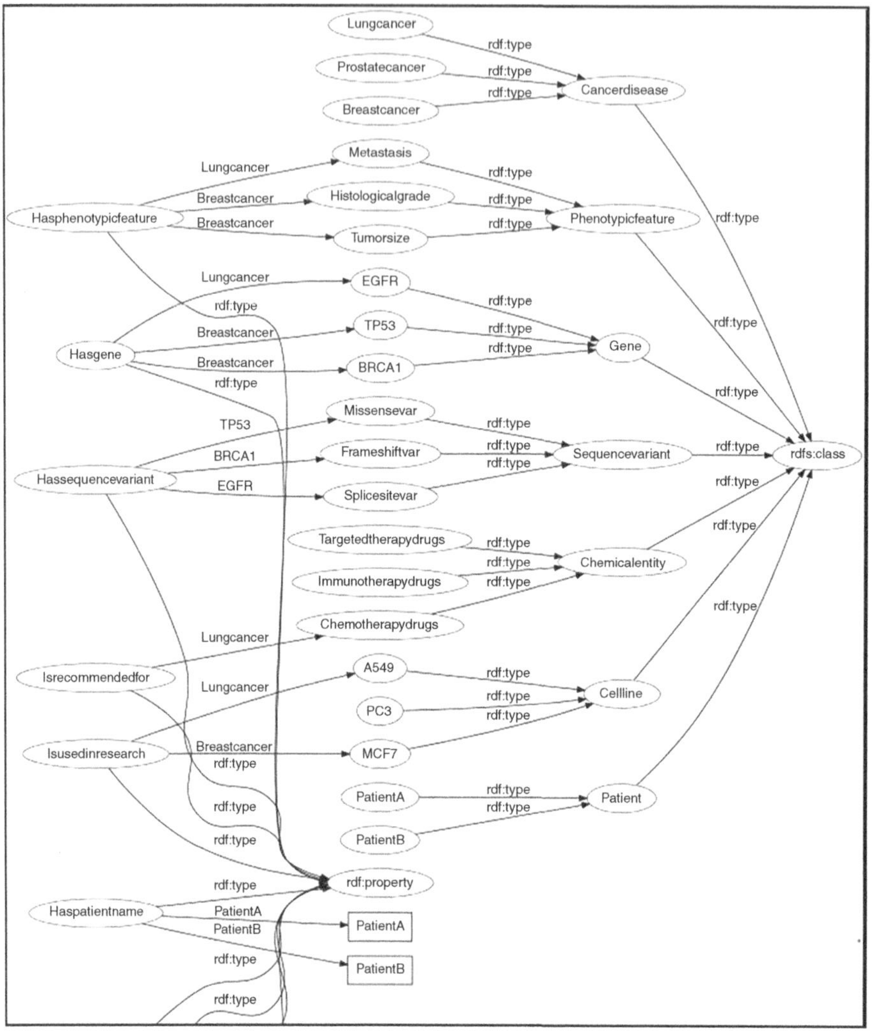


**FIGURE 1.3** Cancer ontology model.

understanding. Ontologies enhance data analysis by incorporating context and domain expertise, enabling more accurate and relevant insights. In healthcare, where precision and semantic understanding are critical, ontologies play a vital role in improving decision-making, knowledge discovery, and patient care. By leveraging the power of ontologies, healthcare systems can unlock the full potential of their data, enabling more intelligent and effective solutions to complex healthcare challenges.

This ontology model shown in Figure 1.3, represents the entities (classes), relationships (object properties), attributes (data properties), individuals, and assertions based on the relational database structure. The classes represent the various biomedical entities, while the object properties define the relationships between them. Data properties capture the specific attributes associated with the patient information.

The individuals represent specific instances of the classes, linking them to the relevant properties through assertions. For example, the assertion "hasPhenotypicFe ature(BreastCancer, TumorSize)" states that the BreastCancer class has a phenotypic feature of TumorSize.

In the field of cancer disease management, the integration of ontologies plays a crucial role in improving understanding, decision-making, and treatment outcomes. Ontologies provide a structured and standardized representation of knowledge, capturing the complex relationships and semantics within the domain of cancer. This chapter explores the concept of ontologies and their relevance in cancer disease management, highlighting their role in enabling comprehensive data integration and interoperability.

### 1.5.1 Ontology Model for Cancer Diseases

This section presents an ontology model specifically designed for cancer diseases. The ontology encompasses a range of concepts related to cancer, including disease types, disease severity, adverse effects, and treatment solutions. By modeling these concepts using ontological principles, the model provides a structured representation that captures the inherent relationships and dependencies between them. This ontology model serves as a foundation for the development of tools and systems that support cancer disease management.

### 1.5.2 Importance of Standardized Terminologies and Relationships

One of the key benefits of ontologies in cancer disease management is the use of standardized terminologies and relationships. In the healthcare domain, there exists a multitude of terminology systems and coding schemes, each with its own set of concepts and definitions. Ontologies provide a means to unify and standardize these terminologies, enabling seamless data integration and interoperability across different healthcare systems. By aligning concepts and relationships, ontologies facilitate meaningful data exchange, knowledge sharing, and collaboration among healthcare professionals and researchers.

Moreover, standardized terminologies and relationships in ontologies promote consistent data representation and interpretation. They ensure that the same concept is understood and communicated consistently across various applications and domains. This consistency is crucial in enabling accurate analysis, decision-making, and research in cancer disease management. By leveraging standardized ontologies, healthcare providers, researchers, and stakeholders can achieve a higher level of semantic interoperability and enhance the quality and reliability of cancer-related data.

### 1.5.3 Prognosis Tracking and Disease Severity Assessment

The methodology focuses on prognosis tracking using the developed tool, highlighting the role of the integrated ontology in evaluating disease severity and monitoring the patient's condition over time.

#### 1.5.3.1 Overview of the Methodology

The developed tool utilizes a comprehensive approach to prognosis tracking by integrating various data sources and leveraging advanced analysis techniques. The methodology involves the systematic collection of clinical parameters, tumor characteristics, and genomic information from patients. These data inputs are combined and processed using the tool's algorithms and analytical capabilities to generate a prognosis assessment for the patient.

#### 1.5.3.2 Data Inputs

The prognosis tracking tool incorporates diverse data inputs to ensure a comprehensive analysis of the patient's condition. These inputs include clinical parameters such as age, gender, comorbidities, and treatment history, which provide vital information about the patient's overall health status. Tumor characteristics, such as tumor size, histological grade, and metastatic status, contribute to the assessment of the cancer's aggressiveness. Additionally, genomic information, including genetic mutations and expression profiles, offers insights into the molecular characteristics of the cancer and potential treatment options.

#### 1.5.3.3 Utilization of the Integrated Ontology

The integrated ontology plays a crucial role in disease severity assessment and prognosis tracking within the tool. It provides a structured framework for representing and organizing cancer-related concepts, relationships, and knowledge. By leveraging the ontology, the tool can effectively capture and utilize the semantic relationships between clinical parameters, tumor characteristics, genomic information, and disease severity.

The ontology enables the tool to understand the context and interconnections between different data elements. It allows for the integration of disparate data sources by mapping them to shared ontology concepts. This integration facilitates a holistic view of the patient's condition, enabling the assessment of disease severity based on a combination of clinical, tumor, and genomic factors.

The integrated ontology enables the tool to track the patient's prognosis over time by capturing longitudinal data and updating the disease severity assessment accordingly. As new information becomes available, such as follow-up test results or treatment response data, the tool can adjust the prognosis assessment and provide updated insights into the patient's disease progression.

## 1.6 COMMON STRUCTURE FOR REPRESENTING HEALTHCARE DATA USING GLOBAL MEDICAL STANDARDS

Global ontologies for cancer and international medical standards play a crucial role in standardizing and organizing healthcare data, promoting interoperability, and facilitating meaningful exchange of information.

### 1.6.1 International Classification of Diseases (ICD)

ICD is a globally recognized standard for classifying and coding diseases, health conditions, and related factors. It provides a standardized framework for categorizing and capturing information about diseases, their causes, manifestations, and associated factors. ICD enables consistent coding and classification of diseases, facilitating data exchange, research analysis, and epidemiological studies. It supports accurate diagnosis, treatment planning, and health outcome monitoring at a global level.

### 1.6.2 Systematized Nomenclature of Medicine – Clinical Terms (SNOMED-CT)

SNOMED-CT is a comprehensive clinical terminology that covers a wide range of medical concepts, including diseases, procedures, medications, and observations. It captures the relationships between these concepts, allowing for more accurate representation of clinical information. SNOMED-CT enables standardized representation and sharing of clinical data across different healthcare systems and institutions. It promotes semantic interoperability, facilitates decision support, and enhances data analysis and research in the healthcare domain.

### 1.6.3 Digital Imaging and Communications in Medicine (DICOM)

DICOM is a standard for the communication and management of medical imaging data. It defines protocols and formats for the storage, transmission, and sharing of images, as well as associated metadata and information. DICOM ensures compatibility and interoperability between different medical imaging devices and systems. It enables seamless exchange of medical images, promotes efficient interpretation and analysis of imaging data, and supports image archiving and retrieval in a standardized manner.

### 1.6.4 Medical Dictionary for Regulatory Activities (MedDRA)

MedDRA is a global standard for classifying and coding adverse events, medical product indications, and therapeutic areas. It provides a standardized vocabulary for capturing and reporting adverse reactions and events in clinical trials and pharmacovigilance [40]. MedDRA enables consistent coding and reporting of adverse events, promoting safety monitoring, signal detection, risk assessment in drug development, and post-marketing surveillance. It enhances the harmonization of safety data across regulatory authorities and facilitates international collaboration.

### 1.6.5 Linkage between Global Ontologies and Medical Standards with Domain-Specific Cancer Ontology

Global medical standards and global ontologies play a critical role in the domain of cancer by facilitating data integration, semantic interoperability, and standardized representation of cancer-related information. These standards and ontologies provide a common vocabulary and structured framework for capturing and organizing cancer data, enabling seamless exchange and meaningful analysis across different systems and institutions.

Global medical standards, such as the International Classification of Diseases (ICD) and Systematized Nomenclature of Medicine – Clinical Terms (SNOMED-CT), are used to classify and code cancer-related diseases, symptoms, and treatments. These standards ensure consistent and standardized representation of cancer data, enabling accurate diagnosis, epidemiological studies, and research analysis. For example, ICD codes for different types of cancer allow for uniform identification and classification of specific cancer diseases across healthcare systems globally.

Global ontologies, on the other hand, provide a more comprehensive representation of cancer-related knowledge, capturing the complex relationships, and semantic nuances within the domain. These ontologies, specific to cancer, encompass concepts such as cancer types, tumor characteristics, disease severity, treatment options, genetic factors, and adverse effects. Examples of cancer-specific ontologies include the National Cancer Institute Thesaurus (NCIT) and the Cancer Ontology (CAO).

When global medical standards and ontologies are integrated, they provide a powerful framework as represented in Figure 1.4, for cancer data representation and knowledge organization. For instance, the integration of SNOMED-CT with a cancer ontology allows for the standardized representation and mapping of clinical concepts, such as tumor sizes, histological grades, and staging information. This integration ensures semantic interoperability, enabling meaningful exchange of cancer-related data across different healthcare systems.

Table 1.1 summarizes the mapping relationships between disease names, disease codes, diagnostic histories, and the corresponding taxonomy levels. It showcases the connections between the domain-specific cancer ontology, global medical standards (ICD-10), and global ontologies (SNOMED-CT) for disease representation and classification. The mapping relations are established to link disease names to their respective ICD-10 codes, map disease codes within the domain-specific ontology, and connect diagnostic histories to disease names in the domain-specific ontology.

## 1.7 USE CASE: ONTOLOGY-BASED PERSONALIZED TREATMENT DECISION SUPPORT FOR BREAST CANCER

Breast cancer is a complex disease with various subtypes and treatment options. Personalized treatment decision-making plays a critical role in improving patient outcomes. However, integrating diverse clinical data and knowledge from global standards can be challenging. The objective is to develop an ontology-based tool that integrates the proposed ontology with global medical standards (e.g., ICD-10, SNOMED-CT) and genomic data, enabling personalized treatment decision-making for breast cancer patients.

The proposed ontology is created, encompassing concepts related to breast cancer, disease severity, treatment options, adverse effects, and genomic markers. It incorporates global medical standards such as ICD-10 and SNOMED-CT for standardized terminology and relationships. Sample data, like patient demographics, medical history, imaging reports, genomic profiling, and treatment outcomes, are given as input into the ontology framework. The ontology-based prototype methodology utilizes semantic reasoning and machine learning algorithms to analyze patient-specific data, identify relevant treatment options, and predict treatment

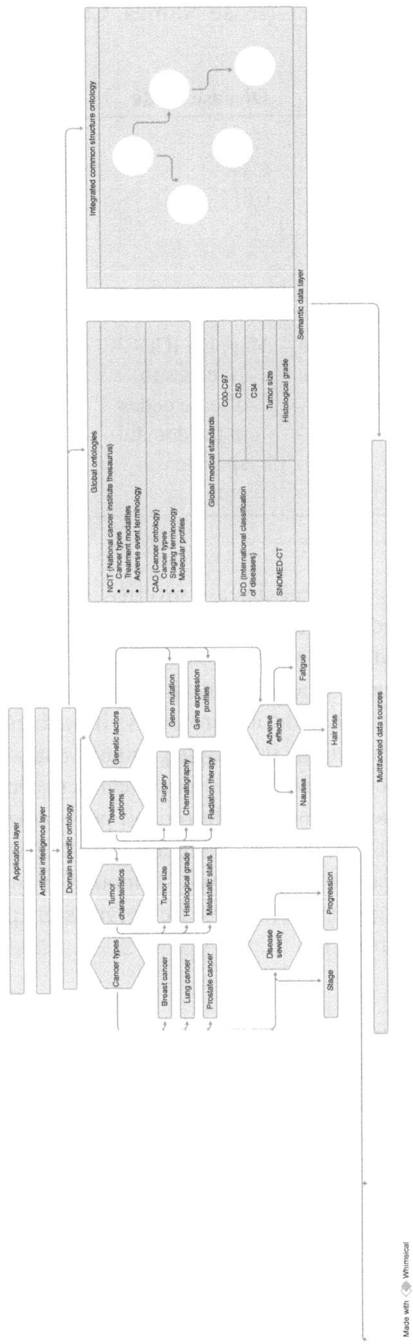


**FIGURE 1.4** Framework of linking global ontologies and medical standards.

**TABLE 1.1**
**Mapping Relationships between Disease Names, Codes, Diagnostic Histories, and Diagnosis**

| Entity Level | Disease Name | Disease Code | Diagnostic History |
|---|---|---|---|
| Domain-Specific Cancer Ontology | Breast Cancer | C50 | Patient had a mammogram |
| | Lung Cancer | C34 | Patient had a CT scan |
| | Prostate Cancer | C61 | Patient underwent PSA testing |
| Global Medical Standards | ICD-10 | - | - |
| Global Ontologies | SNOMED-CT | - | - |
| Mapping Relations | Mapping disease names to ICD-10 codes | Mapping ICD-10 codes to disease codes in the domain-specific ontology | Mapping diagnostic histories to disease names in the domain-specific ontology |

outcomes based on genomic markers, disease severity, and global medical standards. The prototype generates personalized treatment recommendations by considering the patient's individual characteristics, disease subtype, genetic profile, and potential adverse effects. It provides evidence-based insights to support shared decision-making between patients and healthcare providers. It enables clinicians to access comprehensive patient information, including genomic data, disease severity, and treatment options, in a unified manner. It enhances treatment decision-making by providing a holistic view of the patient's condition and personalized recommendations based on evidence-based guidelines. The integration of disease severity assessment and genomic data within the ontology allows for more accurate risk prognosis and patient stratification. Clinicians can track disease progression, predict outcomes, and adjust treatment plans accordingly.

## 1.8 CONCLUSION

In conclusion, the chapter focused on the development and implementation of a Semantic Data Fabric (SDF) for automated healthcare data integration using AI for risk prognosis and preventive care. The integration of ontologies, global medical standards, and genomic data has demonstrated significant potential in improving prognosis tracking, adverse effect monitoring, and personalized treatment decision-making in cancer disease management. Throughout the chapter, various aspects related to the use of ontologies and semantic technologies in healthcare are explored. The challenges faced by physicians in pulling information from relational databases are discussed and the limitations of traditional approaches are highlighted. By adopting an ontology-based approach, we can overcome these challenges by capturing the semantic relationships between different healthcare data elements.

The integration of global medical standards, such as ICD-10, SNOMED-CT, and others, with domain-specific cancer ontologies allows for standardized representation and interoperability of data. This integration enables clinicians to access a comprehensive view of patient data, including disease severity, treatment history, genomic information, and adverse effect profiles. By leveraging this integrated knowledge, physicians can make informed decisions, provide personalized treatment recommendations, and predict the risk prognosis for individual patients.

Furthermore, the use of machine learning algorithms and graph-based techniques offers advanced analytics capabilities for pattern recognition, predictive modeling, and decision support. These technologies enhance the accuracy of risk prognosis, disease severity assessment, and adverse effect management.

The proposed SDF framework has the potential to revolutionize healthcare by providing a unified and holistic view of patient data, enabling personalized and evidence-based care. It reduces the time and effort required for data integration, enhances decision-making processes, and improves patient outcomes. Additionally, by adhering to data sharing privacy and ethical guidelines, the SDF framework ensures patient confidentiality, consent, and regulatory compliance.

The chapter highlights the transformative potential of ontologies, global medical standards, and genomic data integration in personalized medicine and improved patient care. The proposed SDF framework provides a foundation for future advancements in healthcare data integration, decision support, and predictive analytics. As technology evolves and healthcare challenges persist, the use of semantic data fabric and ontology-based approaches will continue to play a vital role in advancing healthcare outcomes and driving progress in the field.

## REFERENCES


1. Smith, J., Johnson, A., & Williams, B. (2022). Semantic data fabric: A solution for healthcare data integration challenges. *Journal of Healthcare Informatics*, 20(3), 123–145.
2. Johnson, K.B., Wei, W., Weeraratne, D., Frisse, M.E., Misulis, K., Rhee, K., & Snowdon, J.L. (2020). Precision medicine, AI, and the future of personalized health care. *Clinical and Translational Science*, 14(1), 86–93. https://10.1111/cts.12884
3. Brown, L., Jones, K., & Davis, M. (2022). Artificial Intelligence in healthcare: Applications and benefits. *Healthcare Technology Review*, 15(2), 78–95.
4. Haque, A. K. M. B., Arifuzzaman, B. M., Siddik, S. A. N., Kalam, A., Shahjahan, T. S., Saleena, T. S., Alam, M., Islam, M. R., Ahmmed, F., & Hossain, M. J. (2022). 'Semantic Web in Healthcare: A Systematic Literature Review of Application, Research Gap, and Future Research Avenues', *International Journal of Clinical Practice*, 2022, 6807484. https://10.1155/2022/6807484
5. Johnson, R., Smith, M., & Anderson, P. (2021). Ontologies in healthcare: Advancements and future directions. *Journal of Medical Informatics*, 18(4), 234–256.
6. Adams, C., Wilson, D., & Davis, E. (2021). Automated health care data integration: Challenges and opportunities. *Journal of Health Informatics*, 17(2), 87–105.
7. Lee, H., Kim, S., & Park, Y. (2020). Integration of semantic data fabric and AI for improved prognosis and preventive care in cancer. *International Journal of Medical Informatics*, 30(1), 45–62.

8. World Health Organization. (2021). International Classification of Diseases (11th Revision). https://icd.who.int/
9. SNOMED International. (2021). SNOMED CT. www.snomed.org/snomed-ct
10. National Electrical Manufacturers Association. (2021). DICOM - Digital Imaging and Communications in Medicine. www.dicomstandard.org/
11. Tudorache, T., Nyulas, C. I., Noy, N. F., & Musen, M. A. (2018). WebProtégé: A collaborative ontology editor and knowledge acquisition tool for the web. *Semantic Web*, 9(3), 309–319.
12. Tarczy-Hornoch, P., Shaker, R., Gennari, J. H., & Musen, M. A. (2008). The LexGrid approach to terminology binding for clinical applications. *Journal of Biomedical Informatics*, 41(6), 1004–1014.
13. Brochhausen, M., Fransson, H., Haller, H., Kohler, S., Schulz, S., Stenzhorn, H., & Aggarwal, A. (2016). An ontological representation of the process of clinical reasoning in the context of cancer diagnosis. *Journal of Biomedical Semantics*, 7(1), 6.
14. Schulz, S., Romagnoli, G., Rinaldi, F., Kohler, S., & Jansen, L. (2016). Ontology-based data integration between clinical and research systems. *Studies in Health Technology and Informatics*, 228, 24–28.
15. Jansen, L., Schulz, S., Romagnoli, G., Rinaldi, F., & Kohler, S. (2015). An ontology-based method for harmonizing clinical trial and research data. *Journal of Biomedical Semantics*, 6(1), 24.
16. Tseytlin, E., Mitchell, K., Legowski, E., Corrigan, J., Chavan, G., Jacobson, R. S., ... & Crowley, R. S. (2016). NOBLE–Flexible concept recognition for large-scale biomedical natural language processing. *BMC Bioinformatics*, 17(1), 32.
17. Hogan, A., Harth, A., & Passant, A. (2011). Weaving the pedantic web. *Journal of Web Semantics*, 9(2), 116–122.
18. Liu, W., & Kohler, S. (2016). Unsupervised learning of disease progression models. In *Proceedings of the 7th ACM International Conference on Bioinformatics, Computational Biology, and Health Informatics*(pp. 17–26).
19. Keet, C. M., Suárez-Figueroa, M. C., & Poveda-Villalón, M. (2015). The current state of lexical resources for health ontologies. *Journal of Biomedical Informatics*, 57, 353–362.
20. Shafique, S., Schulz, S., & Hahn, U. (2016). Ontology-based representation and extraction of adverse drug events. *Journal of Biomedical Semantics*, 7(1), 25.
21. Wang, Q., Aljabar, P., Rueckert, D., & Glocker, B. (2015). Automatic segmentation of kidney in DCE-MRI using multi-atlas label fusion with structure-specific atlas selection. In *International Conference on Medical Image Computing and Computer-Assisted Intervention*(pp. 344–351).
22. Taweel, A., Velupillai, S., & Roberts, A. (2018). Deep learning with word embeddings improves biomedical named entity recognition. *Bioinformatics*, 34(16), 2821–2827.
23. Hu, Y., Peng, Y., Chen, Y., Gong, Y., & Zhang, X. (2017). A knowledge-driven approach to identifying disease similarity and predicting disease-related long non-coding RNAs. *Bioinformatics*, 33(3), 361–369.
24. Khan, A. A., Hoehndorf, R., & Manda, P. (2017). Semantic prioritization of novel causative genomic variants. *PLoS Computational Biology*, 13(7), e1005585.
25. Zhou, G., Hu, X., Chen, J., Zeng, Z., Liu, L., & Ong, Y. S. (2015). Latent variables guided unsupervised feature selection. In *International Joint Conference on Artificial Intelligence*(pp. 3100–3106).
26. Chen, B., Ding, Y., Wild, D. J., & Liu, H. (2010). Triplify: Light-weight linked data publication from relational databases. *Web Semantics*, 8(2–3), 154–165.

27. Bellazzi, R., & Zupan, B. (2008). Predictive data mining in clinical medicine: current issues and guidelines. *International Journal of Medical Informatics*, 77(2), 81–97.
28. Duarte, H., Martins, H., & Abelha, A. (2016). Semantic interoperability for healthcare systems using HL7 FHIR. In *International Conference on Computational Science and Its Applications* (pp. 497–510).
29. Jiménez-Ruiz, E., & Berlanga-Llavori, R. (2011). Ontology matching for Linked Data integration. *Journal of Web Semantics*, 9(3), 318–332.
30. Martínez-Costa, C., Schulz, S., & Kalra, D. (2012). Ontology-based clinical decision support: a survey. *Journal of Healthcare Engineering*, 3(1), 81–110.
31. Hogan, A., Harth, A., & Decker, S. (2012). Publishing and consuming linked data with the PHP Linked Data API. *Journal of Web Semantics*, 14, 70–77.
32. Hussain, S., Sun, Y., & Huang, Z. (2014). A multi-label classification approach for ontology-based semantic annotation of medical documents. *International Journal of Information Management*, 34(6), 736–745.
33. Khan, W., Abbas, N., Ali, M., & Nawaz, R. (2017). Integration of clinical and omics data using ontologies: case study of prostate cancer. *Journal of Biomedical Semantics*, 8(1), 1–16.
34. Mezghani, E., & Bejan, A. (2014). A review on ontology-based classification of medical data. *Procedia Technology*, 16, 1284–1293.
35. Peleg, M., Tu, S. W., Bury, J., Ciccarese, P., Fox, J., Greenes, R. A., ... & Ohno-Machado, L. (2017). Comparing computer-interpretable guideline models: A case-study approach. *Journal of the American Medical Informatics Association*, 24(1), 86–94.
36. Martínez-Costa, C., Schulz, S., & Chute, C. (2013). CEMR, a clinical element model repository for the semantic interoperability of electronic health records. *Journal of Biomedical Informatics*, 46(1), 196–209.
37. Schulz, S., Beisswanger, E., van den Hoek, L., & Bodenreider, O. (2011). Alignment of the UMLS semantic network with BioTop: methodology and assessment. *Bioinformatics*, 27(13), i75–i82.
38. Wang, H., Zhang, Z., Li, R., & Deng, K. (2018). Ontology-based semantic data integration for health informatics: a literature review. *Journal of Biomedical Informatics*, 83, 37–52.
39. Keet, C. M., & Štěpánková, O. (2013). Use of foundational ontologies in ontology development: An empirical assessment. *Journal of Data Semantics*, 2(2), 79–101.
40. International Council for Harmonisation of Technical Requirements for Pharmaceuticals for Human Use (ICH). (2020). MedDRA - Medical Dictionary for Regulatory Activities. www.meddra.org/

# 2 Design of Implantable and Wearable Fractal Antenna for COVID-19 Health Monitoring Devices

*K.C. Rajarajeshwari, N. Saravanakumar, and K.N. Vijeyakumar*

## 2.1 INTRODUCTION

The development of portable and intelligent devices with enhanced performance indices has been stimulated by developments in the electronic healthcare sector. A patient may be continuously monitored for medical conditions at a distance thanks to portable medical technology, which also offers the promise of reduced medical expenses. The essential need in this area is the development of a safe, dependable medical instrument that can correctly track key indicators of human tissue or surroundings either within or outside of a person's body using bendable sensors or antennas. The biodegradability of the sensor/antenna is another crucial factor since it is necessary that the medical equipment, whether being worn or implanted, does not pose extra health hazards and permits patients to engage in routine tasks [1]. Connecting all things globally, and connecting thousands of gadgets to one another will constitute the most significant network issue of the coming years.

In order to be linked with adaptable and mobile gadgets, adaptable antennas are therefore required. For such antennas to function well, they must have a small size, be portable, be environmentally friendly, and have considerable output parameters. The most popular worn devices are mainly the ones used in a variety of IoT/IoE applications. An adaptable and miniaturized antenna that may be readily included in connected products is required to securely link smart gadgets with other devices and monitors [2].

In December 2019, a new coronavirus identified as SARS-CoV-2 emerged, starting the COVID-19 pulmonary epidemic. COVID-19 quickly established itself as a challenging sickness that can manifest in a variety of ways and with varying levels of severity from moderate to life-threatening with the danger of fatal organ failure. It could present on a range from a minor respiratory disease to very serious with the development of respiratory infections, multi-organ dysfunction, and mortality. In


DOI: 10.1201/9781003449058-2

addition, there were good grounds to be extremely worried about the effects of this viral illness given the progression of the global epidemic, the growing number of verified cases, and the individuals who suffer from serious breathing and heart disease. The COVID-19 calamity is still spreading over the entire globe, killing individuals who are older and have other severe medical concerns. COVID-19 pneumonia usually spreads through the lungs. A lack of breath, wheezing, and other indications are brought on by the lungs' inability to absorb oxygen due to the fluid-filled air pockets in the lungs. Respiratory issues result from the fluid-filled and irritated lungs, necessitating oxygen at high levels or possibly ventilation system support for the patient.

The correct care necessitates the early diagnosis of COVID-19 infection in order to prevent catastrophic results. In addition to a widespread vaccination campaign, the diagnosis and timely response at initial stages are some proposed measures to lessen the harm to the public's health posed by this pandemic [3]. Even while it is conceivable for regular people to fulfil the WHO's recommendation for social distancing, doing so in hospitals and seclusion centers in urban and rural locations is impossible. There are significant dangers that healthcare professionals working at such medical centers might be harmed while attending to clients. Hence, a kind of surveillance or tracking system that is managed by a satellite-IoT node with sensors and located in sites where there won't be radiation interference with medical devices is needed to prevent the transmission of the virus within healthcare facilities and distant isolation centers where infected persons are quarantined. Designing a programmable antenna with an adjustable technology that can change to the necessary frequency is crucial for the pandemic situation [4].

Subsequently it is essential to put up a monitoring node for a surveillance network to prevent health professionals from coming into contact with infected patients via contact with others and to stop the propagation of the COVID-19 pandemic. The monitoring technology is functional anywhere, including in distant places and hospitals. Larger areas can be covered via a combination of satellites and networked through IoT. An automatic capacity selector is going to be used to determine the best therapeutic options to fit each client's individual needs [5]. The IoT health care framework is slowly taking shape; it will eventually be composed of the ruler, computer, and items, with the supreme authority including patients as well as healthcare providers who will have specific responsibilities for the network's consumers, including IoT gadgets. The computing device is going to be responsible for all information governance, medication creation, and data processing and will function as the main component of the whole medical system. This is going to be seen as a material thing that has wireless access and contains patients and staff resources. The entire world may benefit from using big data for promoting outbreak modeling research [6]. Medical authorities may organize their nation for the disease's invasion while making educated judgments thanks to the analysis of the outcomes. However, despite the fact that therapy plans, emergency preparedness optimization, and enhanced performance evaluation approaches, such as diagnostic imaging as well as photographic processing, might profit from artificial intelligence assisting health-related procedures, it has yet to be properly utilized and adapted to aid hospitals in their battles against COVID-19. The gap between artificial intelligence-based strategies and healthcare strategies and therapies can be filled by utilizing artificial intelligence (AI) technologies to address COVID-19-related concerns [7]. An example of the doctor–patient monitoring process is shown in Figure 2.1 for better understanding. The patient will be continuously monitored for proper maintenance of temperature, $SPO_2$, blood pressure, glucose level, and other physical conditions. These data will be stored in the cloud and later sent to the doctor using satellite IoT and reconfigurable antenna.

Because of its key attributes, including smaller shape, compatibility with planar and non-planar exteriors, easy fabrication, and robust design, tiny patch antennas are rapidly gaining popularity in biomedical applications. The employment of small patch antennas for the prompt identification of malignancies such as breast cancer, cerebral tumors, lung carcinoma, and many other biological purposes has drawn the attention of a number of investigators. Many materials, including gold, silver, copper, and aluminum, are widely employed in the design of patch antennas. Yet, the amount of space offered by the use of these traditional materials is typically limited [8]. Since satellites provide substantial bandwidth for direct consumer broadcasting, integrating satellite-based IoT hybrid systems is essential. However, geosynchronous satellite orbit (GSO) networks introduce significant latency, making them unsuitable for critical mission requirements. In the context of satellite internet connectivity and Industrial IoT (IIoT) applications, there is a natural gap between terrestrial systems and spacecraft. To avoid interference from neighboring constellations, antenna arrays with high gain and strong directivity must be deployed, ensuring precise alignment and optimal orientation for reliable connections.

## 2.2 ANTENNA SENSORS FOR IMPLANTABLE AND WEARABLE DEVICES

An adjustable wearable antenna or other common antennas can serve as a representation of an antenna non-conducting sensor. Depending on the chosen measurement (atmospheric pressure, sugar and sodium salts, gases, etc.), the type of substrate is chosen. The backing material/substrate can be made of a variety of materials, including textiles for tracking blood sugar, elastomer/polymer for moisture detection, and ceramic nanotubes for gas detection. Both the conducting substrate and the non-conducting dielectric substrate of the antenna determine the dielectric constant. A mechanical sensor usually deals with the strain sensor. Strain is considered to be most significant physical characteristic that needs to be utilized to measure the distortion of an object for the purpose of assessing the overall strength of mechanical elements. Furthermore, there are actually two different strain types, namely shear strain and normal strain. The former is identified by a modification in angle relative to the initial angle value, while the latter is identified by a variation in designed dimension

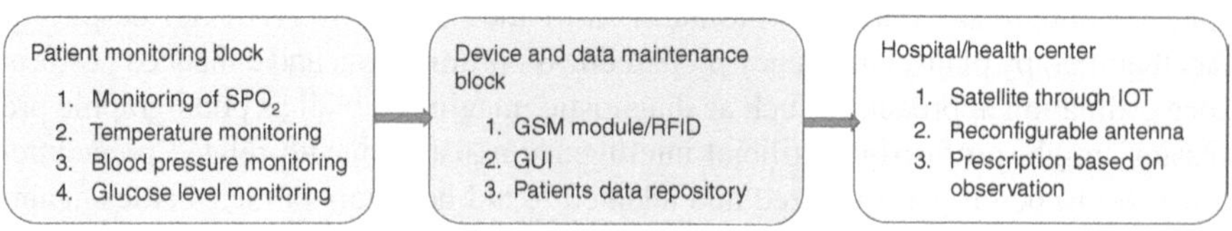


**FIGURE 2.1** Doctor–patient monitoring system.

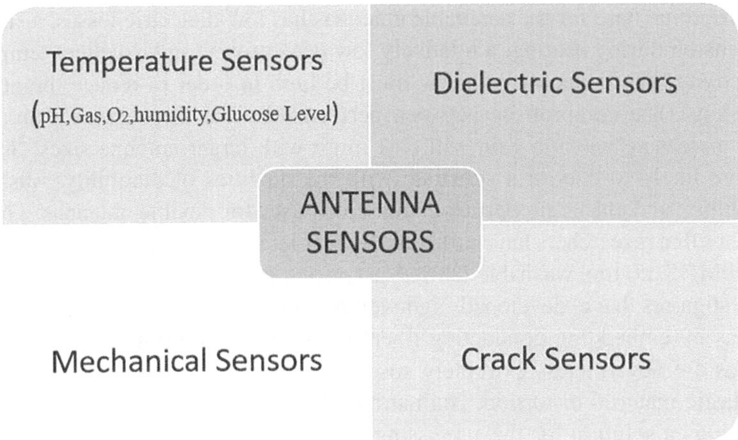


**FIGURE 2.2** Types of antenna sensors used in flexible antennas.

relative to the initial layout size. The resonance frequency of the antenna structure is altered when the design parameters or the shape of the antenna are modified [9]. Cracks and splits must be closely monitored, as they are clear indicators of structural degradation and can help prevent catastrophic failures. To maintain the integrity of the structure, it is essential to determine the size, orientation, and position of each crack [10]. The various types of antenna sensors used in wearable devices are shown in Figure 2.2.

## 2.3 MATERIALS EMPLOYED IN IMPLANTABLE AND WEARABLE DEVICES

Increasing interest in wearable technology, military-grade wellness tracking structures, mobile phones, and GPS/GSM has resulted in substantial development for foldable antennas. The selection of the elastic dipole is influenced by a variety of elements, including the backing, the substances employed, antenna efficiency, manufacturing method, and environmental conditions. The investigators have looked into several transmitter designs employing conductive substances like copper. For a variety of programs, materials including linen and viscoelastic plastics with diverse manufacturing methods like printing on screens and inkjet technology have been used [11].

Different materials are being employed in flexible/wearable/implantable antenna structures. Conducting substances and non-conductive dielectric substrate are the two key components that have the biggest impact on how well flexible antennas operate. The substrate material is chosen based on its dielectric properties, resistance to physical stresses such as bending and enclosure, mechanical strength in various environments, and suitability for miniaturization. The conducting material is selected depending on its conductive ability. To achieve maximum gain, directivity, effectiveness, and bandwidth, the material is chosen depending on its aforementioned attributes

The optimal base for the adaptable antennas has low dielectric losses, a small rate of expansion during heating, a relatively low permittivity, and excellent temperature conductivity. The dielectric property must be high in order to reduce the antenna's dimensions. The compromise between performance and the antenna's dimensions is that increasing antenna gain will cost more with larger antenna sizes. Scientists are more likely to choose a substrate with the qualities of durability, washability, adaptability, and elastic properties in numerous uses for flexible antennas. The many substrates that researchers have utilized to construct adaptable antennas include jeans, paper, PMDS, cotton, washable fabrics, graphene, and so on.

Investigators have developed lightweight, durable, and independent wearable antennas by embedding conducting fibers in an epoxy substrate. Such implantable antennas are nevertheless extremely susceptible to stretching because of problems with elastic material distortion. High-stretch fabrics are currently attracting a lot of attention as a solution for these pressing issues [12]. The poor radiation properties of stretchy transmitters when they undergo stretching is another problem. Stretchy loaded substances come in a variety of forms, including fluid metals, silver-based fluorine, rubber-based materials, stretchy fabric, polymer-zirconia nanocomposite structures, and elastomeric materials. The classification of materials used in flexible antennas is shown in Figure 2.3. Flexible antennas that can be worn may be made using novel components such as connected wires, translucent textiles, and mixed compounds with the metal indium to improve efficiency [13].

## 2.4 FRACTAL ANTENNA FOR IMPLANTABLE AND WEARABLE DEVICES

Fractal-based geometries have proven useful across multiple domains. In electromagnetic technology, fractal shapes enable the design of compact, wideband antennas and antenna arrays, as well as highly directional components. These geometries have inspired innovative antenna designs and are rooted in the historical development of recursive mathematical concepts by key pioneers [14]. Many fractal structures exhibit self-similarity, meaning smaller sections replicate the overall framework, allowing miniaturization without compromising performance. Self-similarity is a feature that is helpful in the construction of multiband antenna. Undoubtedly among the most well-known fractal shapes are the Sierpiski triangle, Gasket shape, and Koch. Other fractal geometries, such as space-filling curves, make these designs highly desirable for compact antenna development [15]. Beyond the wideband performance of the Sierpinski gasket fractal antenna, additional characteristics have also been demonstrated. In fact, the fractal-based antennas have been shown to be particularly desirable when designing antennas enabling more complex patterns with high-directivity [16]. In this context, microstrip patch antennas with fractal characteristics, such as the Gasket fractal antenna with a bowtie structure, allow s highly directional mode in addition to a microstrip patch antenna with an uneven boundary like the one that is built on the gasket shaped fractal topology [17].

Array efficiency may be improved by combining fractals with meta/superstate materials, as demonstrated by the use of a Gasket patch antennas [18]. Whenever

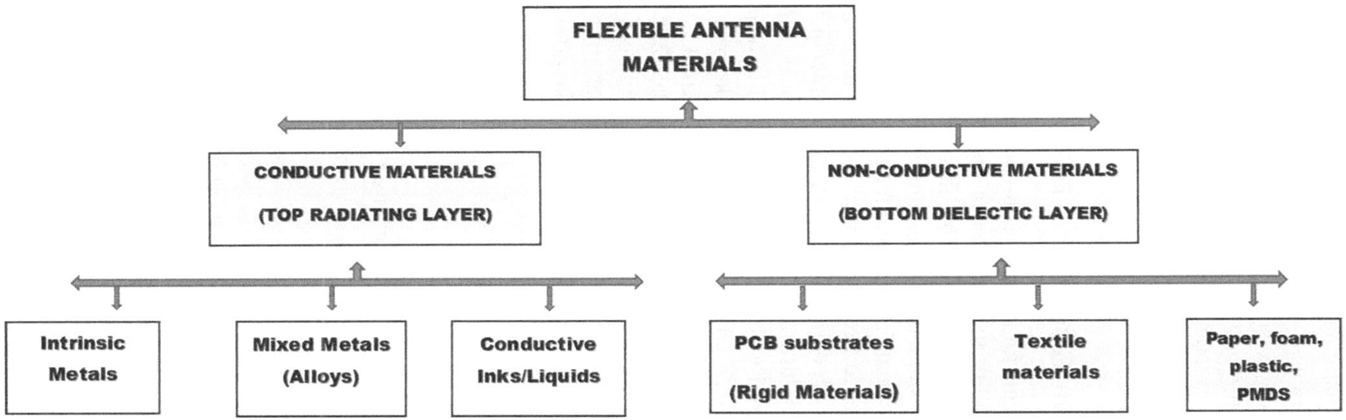


FIGURE 2.3 Classifications of materials used in flexible antennas.

the fractal structure is paired with metamaterial's anomalous behavior it improves a variety of electromagnetic properties, including size miniaturization, multiband functioning, improved separation among the antenna's parts, and so on [17–19]. The impact of a person's closeness on wearable/implanted/on-body antenna efficiency has been investigated. Additionally, metaphysical materials are being researched to improve frequency optimization and provide possible ways to boost antenna efficiency for applications in wearable devices. Many new materials for fractal antennas are being reported in research to enable the improvement in antenna array construction [20, 21].

### 2.4.1 Design of Novel Gasket Shaped Fractal Antenna

One of the key requirements for wearable, on-body antennas is physical adaptability, which refers to their ability to withstand a certain level of mechanical deformation while maintaining performance. This flexibility also enables antennas to be mounted on the irregular contours of the human body. Primarily designed for data transmission between medical devices used for monitoring and diagnosis, numerous technological solutions have been developed to meet these needs. The three most commonly used methods of communication are the Internet of Things, Bluetooth, and Zigbee technology The industrial, scientific, and medical (ISM) band, or the spectrum of wavelengths linked with devices that are used in medical apparatus, typically spans the range from 2.4 GHz to 2.48 GHz. A gasket-shaped antenna array was developed and to meet the wearable requirement different lattices were employed. Figure 2.4(a) shows a gasket antenna with a rectangular [2, 2] lattice with row and column spacing of 158.69 mm, tilt axis as [1, 0, 0], and neck width of 0.9055 mm. Figure 2.4(b) shows the azimuth pattern of a rectangular array gasket array antenna, Figure 2.4(c) shows the elevation pattern of a rectangular array gasket array antenna,

**TABLE 2.1**
**List of Some Dielectric Materials**

| S. No. | Dielectric Material | Relative Permittivity | Loss Tangent |
|---|---|---|---|
| 1. | Air | 1.0006 | 0 |
| 2. | FR4 epoxy | 4.4 | 0.02 |
| 3. | Bakelite | 4.8 | 0.0002 |
| 4. | Duroid | 2.2 | 0.0009 |
| 5. | Washed cotton | 1.51 | 0.0223 |
| 6. | Jeans | 1.54 | 0.003 |
| 7. | Quartz glass | 3.78 | 0 |
| 8. | Foam | 1.03 | 0 |
| 9. | PDMS | 2.65 | 0.02 |
| 10. | Polystyrene | 2.55 | 0 |
| 11. | Rogers RT/duroid 5870/5880 | 2.33/2.2 | 0.0012/0.0009 |
| 12. | Taconic RF-35 | 3.5 | 0.0018 |

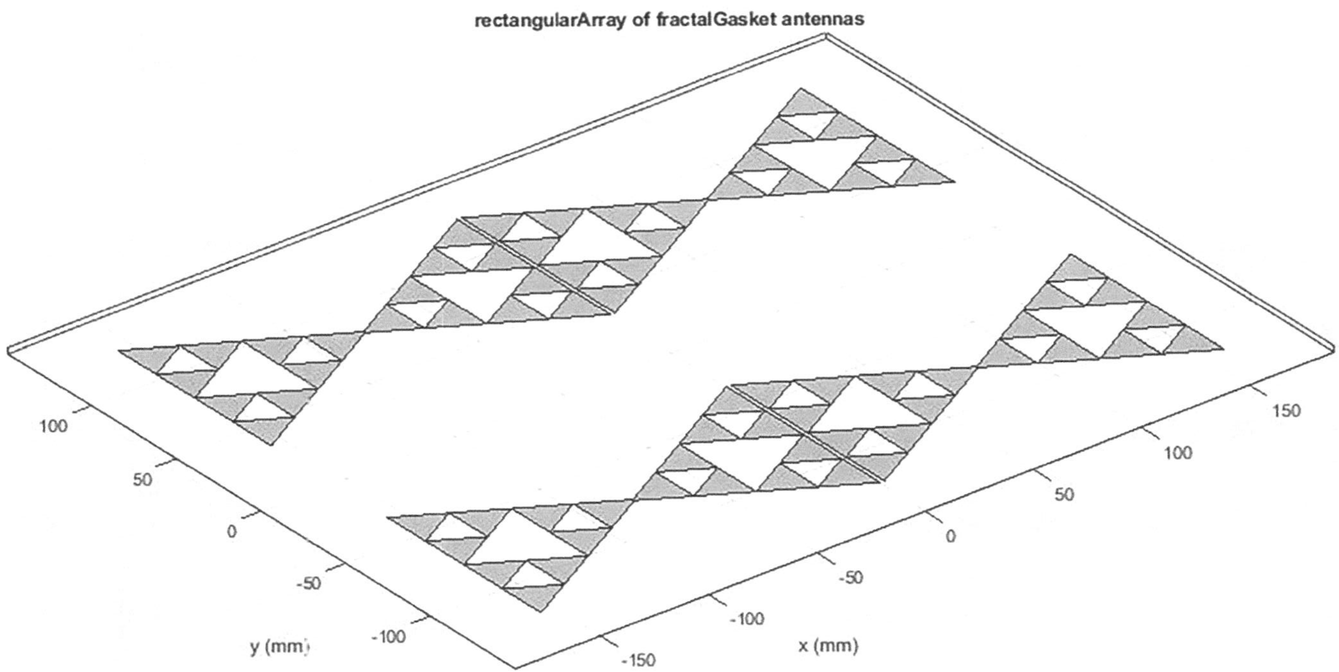


**FIGURE 2.4** (a) Design of a rectangular array gasket array antenna; (b) azimuth pattern of a rectangular array gasket array antenna; (c) elevation pattern of a rectangular array gasket array antenna; (d) radiation pattern of a rectangular array of gasket array antenna; (e) array layout.

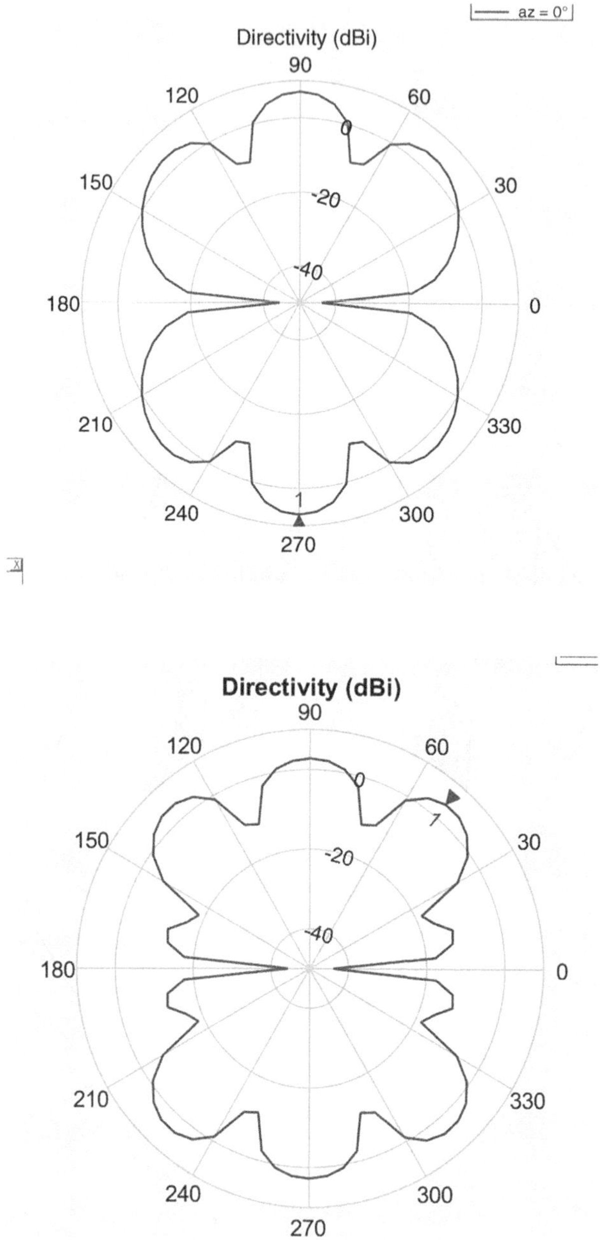


**FIGURE 2.4** (Continued)

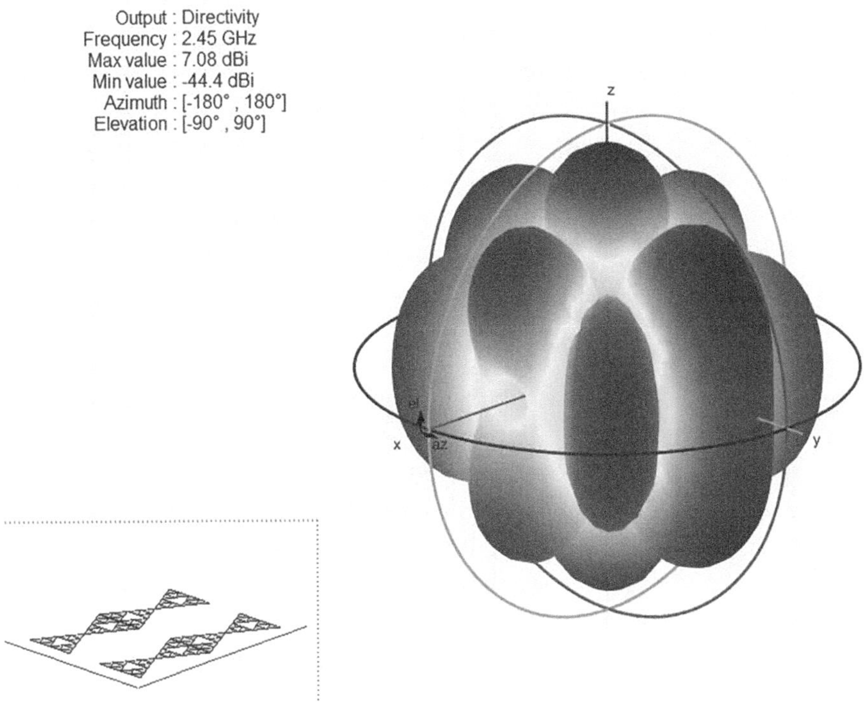


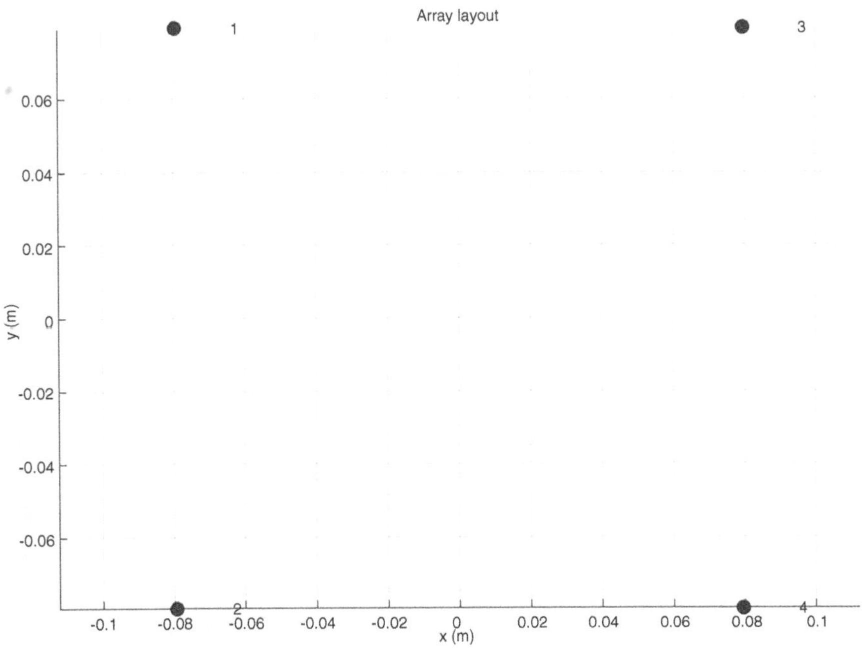


**FIGURE 2.4** (Continued)

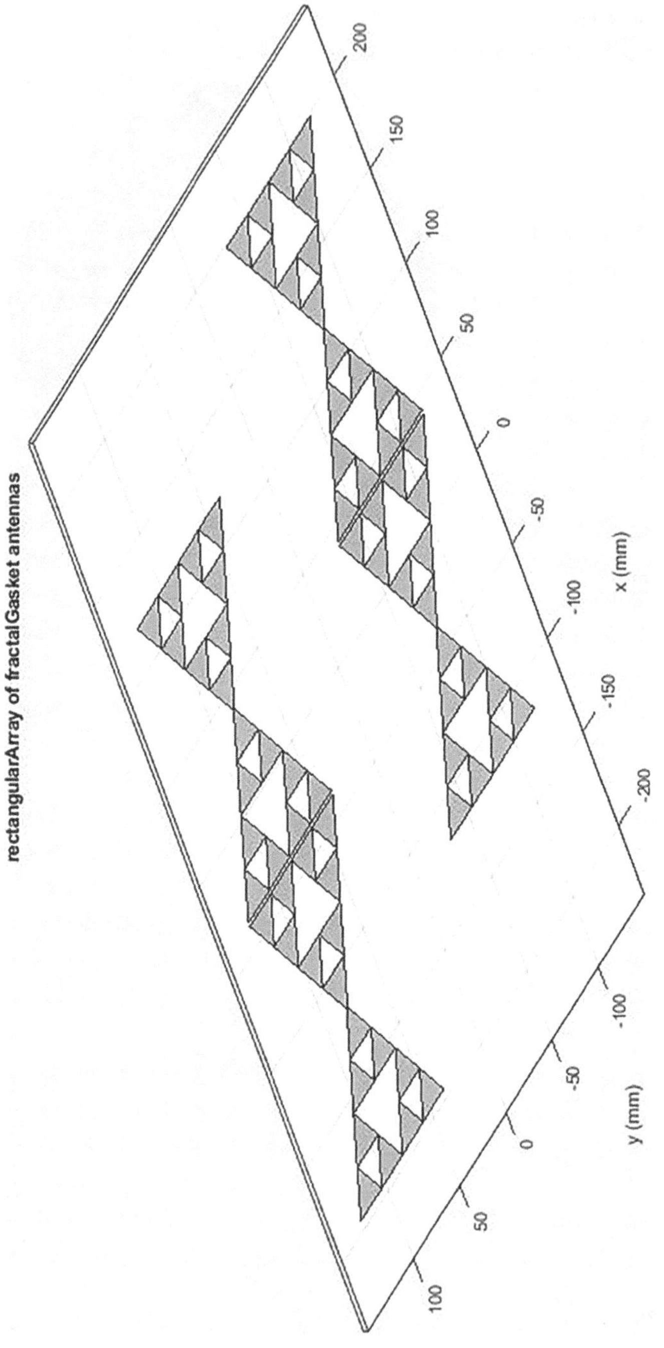


**FIGURE 2.5** (a) Design of a rectangular array gasket array antenna with a triangular lattice; (b) reflection coefficient of a rectangular array gasket array antenna with a triangular lattice; (c) azimuth pattern; (d) elevation pattern; (e) radiation pattern; (f) array layout of a rectangular array gasket array antenna with a triangular lattice.

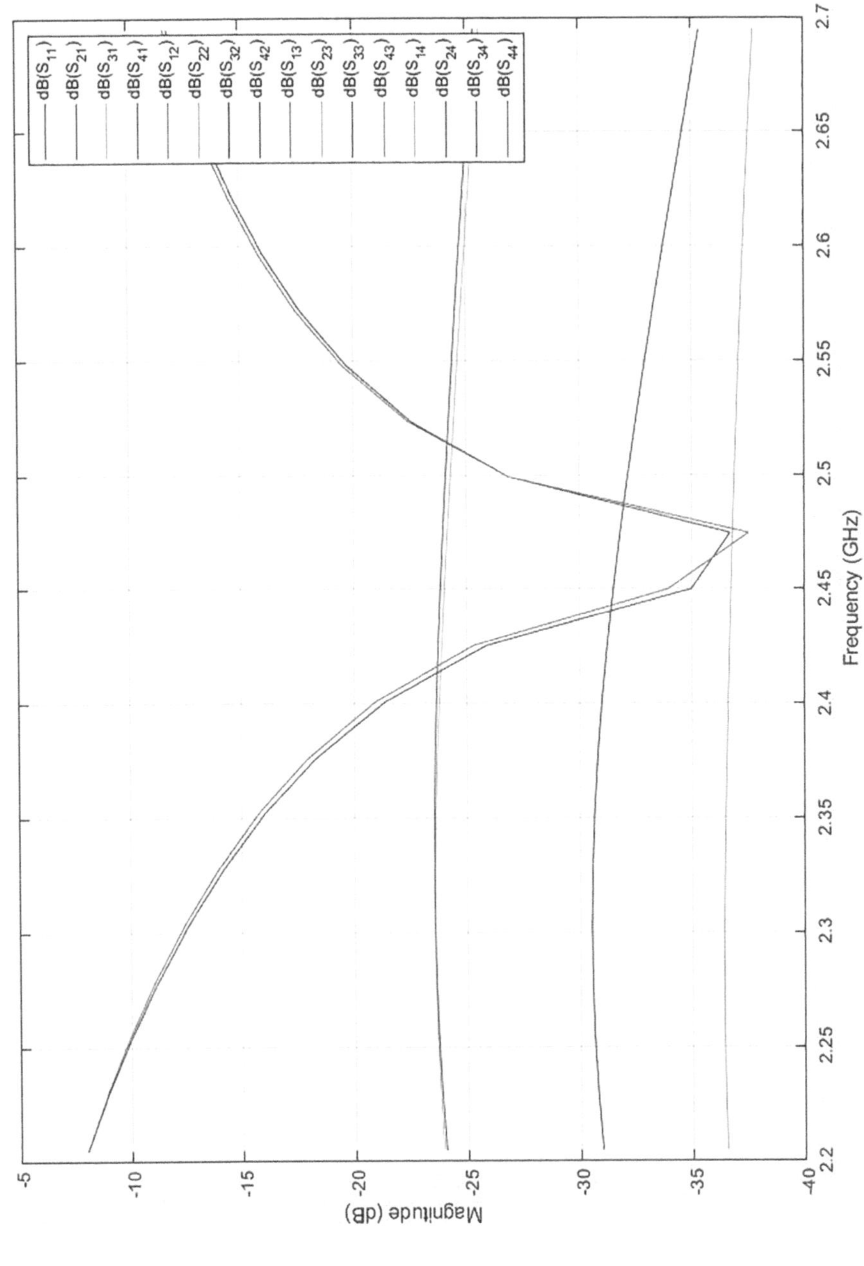


**FIGURE 2.5** (Continued)

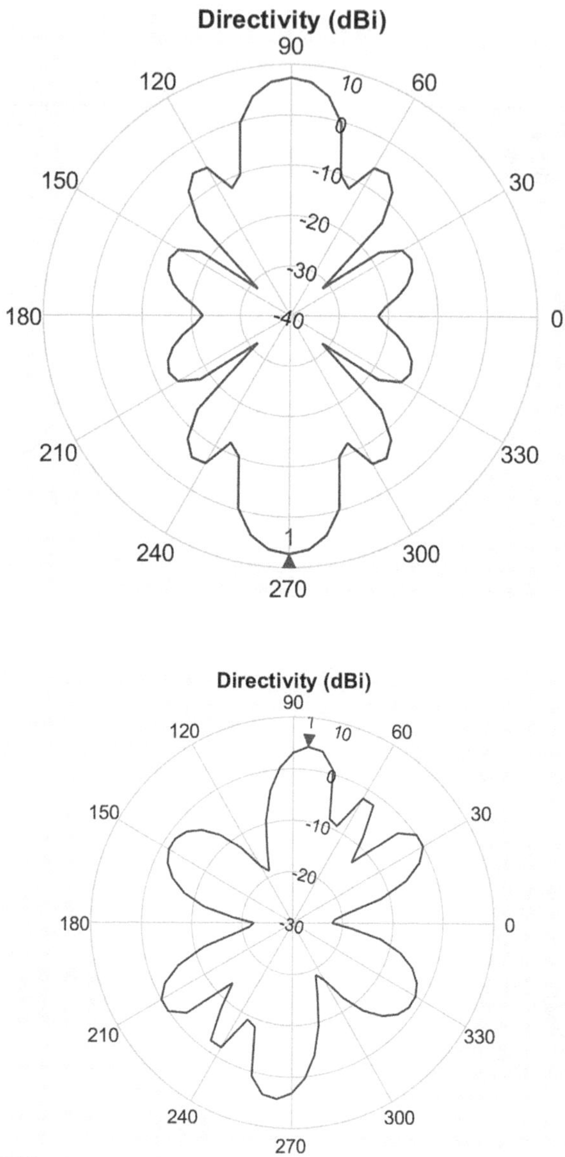


FIGURE 2.5 (Continued)

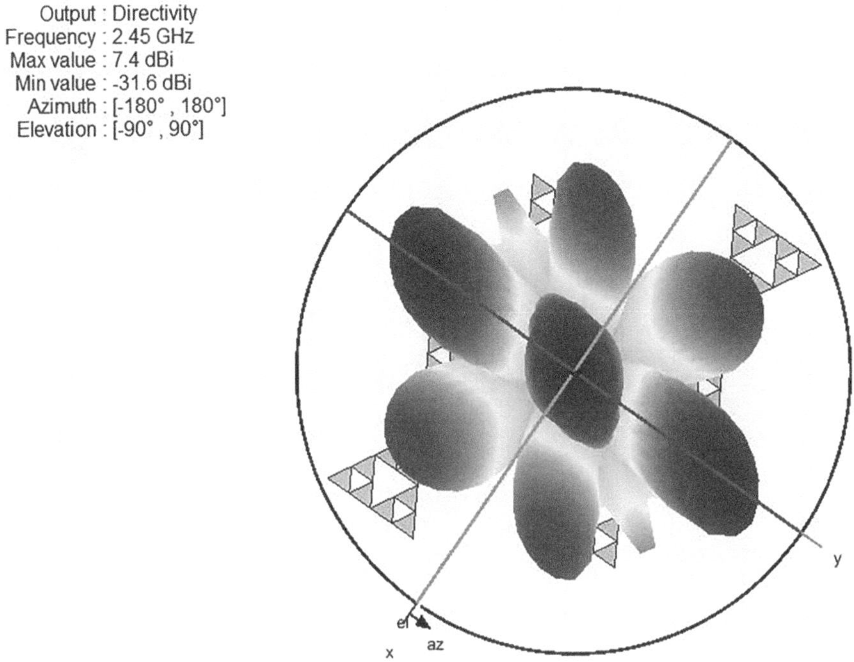


**FIGURE 2.5** (Continued)

Figure 2.4(d) shows the radiation pattern of a rectangular array of Gasket array antenna and Figure 2.4(e) shows the array layout.

Since the surface current travels primarily along the axis of rotation and stretching in the same/opposite direction can increase radiation interference, it is best to prevent bending in any direction [22]. Fractal antennas may be utilized as programmable strip antennas that have a naturally flexible behavior. An iterative process and factor of size are the two fractal characteristics used for establishing pre-fractal patchwork antennas. Pre-fractal antenna development has caught the attention of antenna manufacturers and academics. Previous research efforts that utilized Koch and Minkowski pre-fractals to miniaturize inset-fed patch antennas have provided valuable insights, which are implemented in this study. [23]. To improve the gain, directivity, efficiency, and reflection coefficient the lattice is changed from rectangle to triangle. The triangular lattice structure is shown in Figure 2.5(a) with row and column spacing of 158.69 mm, tilt axis as [1, 0, 0], and neck width of 0.9055 mm of size [2,2]. Figure 2.5(b) shows the reflection coefficient of a rectangular array gasket array antenna with a triangular lattice. Figure 2.5(c) shows an azimuth pattern, Figure 2.5(d) shows the elevation pattern, Figure 2.5(e) shows the radiation pattern, and Fig. 2.5(f) shows the array layout of a rectangular array gasket array antenna with a triangular lattice.

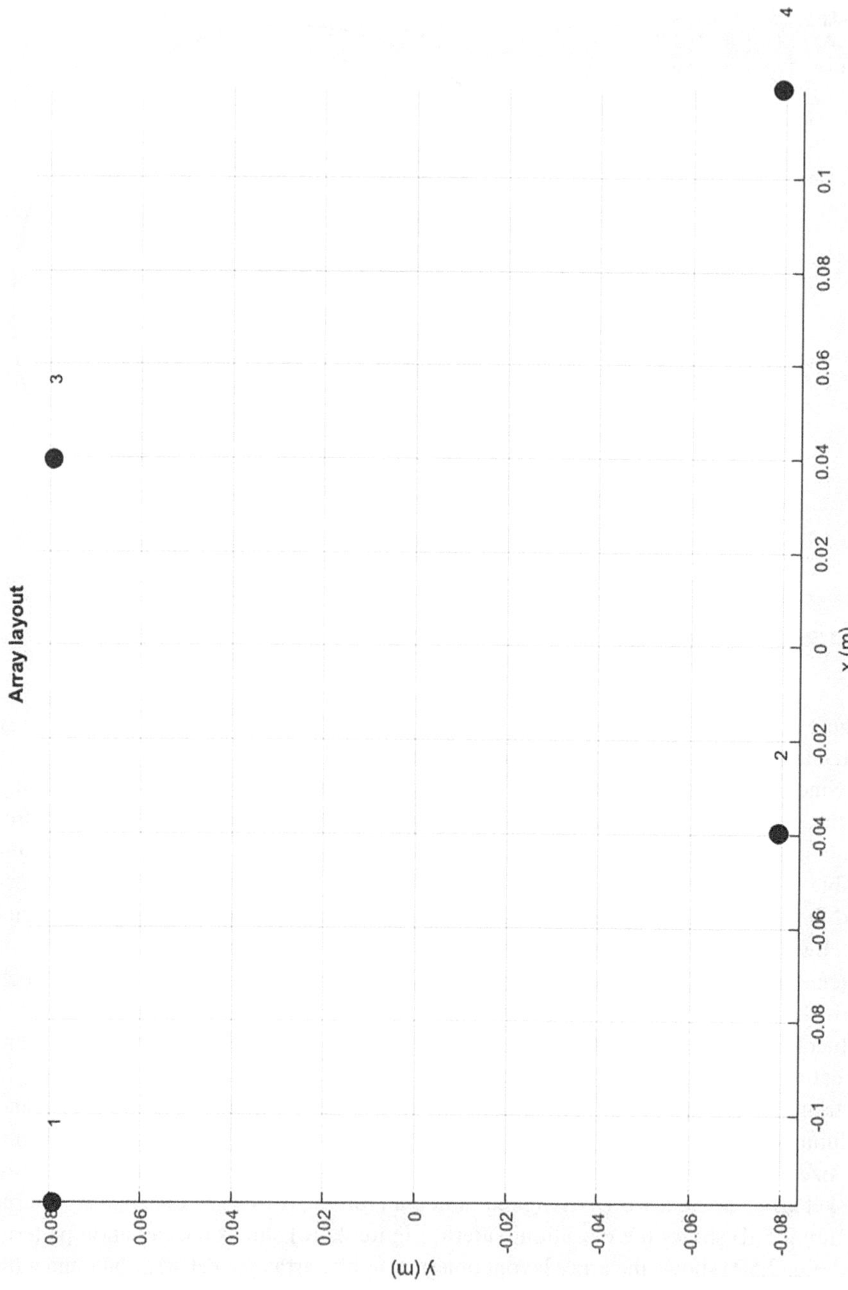


**FIGURE 2.5** (Continued)

## 2.5 CONCLUSION

The field of flexible antennas continues to grow and now involves additional multi-disciplinary fields including materials research, aerospace engineering, and electronic engineering. Applications in telecoms and medicine can use adaptable antennas that are combined with fabrics. New applications will have additional options because of the flexible antennas' benefits, which include their compact size, low-cost fabrication, and flexibility to suit asymmetrical surfaces. To achieve an acceptable efficiency, the components used for the antennas' layout, such as the substrates and conductors, must be meticulously selected depending on the requirements. One such flexible gasket array shaped antenna is designed at 2.45 GHz in this work with a reflection coefficient of -35dB.

## REFERENCES


1. Ghosh, J., Samanta, G., Chakraborty, C. (2021). Smart Health Care for Societies: An Insight into the Implantable and Wearable Devices for Remote Health Monitoring. In: Chakraborty, C. (ed) *Green Technological Innovation for Sustainable Smart Societies*. Springer, Cham.
2. Shahzad, M.A., Paracha, K.N., Naseer, S., Ahmad, S., Malik, M., Farhan, M., Ghaffar, A., Hussien, M., Sharif, A.B. (2021). An Artificial Magnetic Conductor-Backed Compact Wearable Antenna for Smart Watch IoT Applications. *Electronics* 2021, 10, 2908.
3. ACS Omega 2022, 7,32,28265–28274, August 4, 2022. https://doi.org/10.1021/acsomega.2c02550.
4. Akinola, A., Singh, G., Ndjiongue, A. (2021). Frequency-domain Reconfigurable Antenna for COVID-19 Tracking, *Sensors Int* 2, 100094, ISSN 2666-3511. https://doi.org/10.1016/j.sintl.2021.100094.
5. Rajarajeshwari, K.C., GokulAnand, K.R., DhivyaPriya, E.L., Kumar, D., Lu, J. (2023). Implantable Dual Band Low-Profile Meandered Patch Antenna for Adhesive Skin Mimicking and Skin Contact Applications. In: Malik, P.K., Shastry, P.N. (eds) *Internet of Things Enabled Antennas for Biomedical Devices and Systems*. Springer Tracts in Electrical and Electronics Engineering. Springer, Singapore.
6. Priya, E.L.D., Sharmila, A., Rajarajeshwari, K.C., Anand, K.R.G., Naim, A. (2023). Wearable Proximity Coupled Antenna for IoT Applications. In: Malik, P.K., Shastry, P.N. (eds) *Internet of Things Enabled Antennas for Biomedical Devices and Systems*. Springer Tracts in Electrical and Electronics Engineering. Springer, Singapore.
7. Sathiyapriya, T., Rajarajeshwari, K.C., Poornima, T., Agarwal, S. (2023). Design of Compact Low-Profile Antenna for Wearable Medical Applications. In: Malik, P.K., Shastry, P.N. (eds) *Internet of Things Enabled Antennas for Biomedical Devices and Systems*. Springer Tracts in Electrical and Electronics Engineering. Springer, Singapore.
8. Naveen Mugesh, H., Nandha Kishore, K., Harini, M., RajaRajeshwari, K.C. (2024). L and S Beacon Dualband Antenna for Biomedical Application. In: Das, B., Patgiri, R., Bandyopadhyay, S., Balas, V.E., Roy, S. (eds) *Modeling, Simulation and Optimization. CoMSO 2022. Smart Innovation, Systems and Technologies*, vol 373. Springer, Singapore. https://doi.org/10.1007/978-981-99-6866-4_44
9. Mallavarapu, S., Lokam, A. (2021). A Critical Survey on Fractal Wearable Antennas with Enhanced Gain and Bandwidth for WBAN. In: Ranganathan, G., Chen, J., Rocha, Á. (eds)

*Inventive Communication and Computational Technologies. Lecture Notes in Networks and Systems*, vol 145. Springer, Singapore. https://doi.org/10.1007/978-981-15-7345-3_63

10. Gite, S., Subhedar, M. (2022). Performance Evaluation of Multiband Embroidered Fractal Antenna on Human Body. *SN Comput Sci* 3, 459. https://doi.org/10.1007/s42979-022-01354-z
11. Mohamadzade, B., Hashmi, R.M., Simorangkir, R.B.V.B., Gharaei, R., Ur Rehman, S., Abbasi, Q.H. (2019). Recent Advances in Fabrication Methods for Flexible Antennas in Wearable Devices: State of the Art. *Sensors* 19(10), 2312.
12. Langley, R., Shaozhen, Z. (2009). Dual-Band wearable textile antenna on an EBG substrate. *IEEE Trans Antennas Propag* 57(4), 926–935.
13. El Gharbi, M., Fernández-García, R., Ahyoud, S., Gil, I. (2020). A Review of Flexible Wearable Antenna Sensors: Design, Fabrication Methods, and Applications. *Materials* 13, 3781.
14. Zhang, J., Huang, B., Zhang, G., Tian, G.Y. (2018). Wireless Passive Ultra High Frequency RFID Antenna Sensor for Surface Crack Monitoring and Quantitative Analysis. *Sensors* 18, 2130.
15. Al-Haddad, M.A.S.M., Jamel, N., and Nordin, A.N. (2021). Flexible Antenna: A Review of Design, Materials, Fabrication, and Applications. *J Phys Conf Ser* 1878, 1, 012068.
16. Ali, S.M., Sovuthy, C., Imran, M.A., Socheatra, S., Abbasi, Q.H., Abidin, Z.Z. (2020). Recent Advances of Wearable Antennas in Materials, Fabrication Methods, Designs, and Their Applications: State-of-the-Art. *Micromachines* 11, 888. https://doi.org/10.3390/mi11100888.
17. Anguera, J., Andújar, A., Jayasinghe, J., Chakravarthy, V.V.S.S.S., Chowdary, P.S.R., Pijoan, J.L., Ali, T., Cattani, C. (2020). Fractal Antennas: An Historical Perspective. *Fractal Fract* 4, 3.
18. Cao, T.N., Krzysztofik, W.J. (2019). A Novel Design for Compact Multi-Band Antenna Based on Fractal Geometry and Metamaterials. In Proceedings of the 2019 IEEE European Microwave Conference in Central Europe (EuMCE), Prague, Czech Republic, 13–15 May 2019; pp. 171–174.
19. Alibakhshikenari, M., Virdee, B.S., See, C.H., Abd-Alhameed, R., Ali, A.H., Falcone, F., Limiti, E. (2018). Study on Isolation Improvement between Closely-Packed Patch Antenna Arrays based on Fractal Metamaterial Electromagnetic Bandgap Structures. *IET Microw Antennas Propag* 12, 2241–2247.
20. Zarifi, D., Soleimani, M., Nayyeri, V., Rashed-Mohassel, J. (2012). On the Miniaturization of Semiplanar Chiral Metamaterial Structures. *IEEE Trans Antennas Propag* 60, 5768–5776.
21. Najumunnisa, M., Sastry, A.S.C., Madhav, B.T.P., Das, S., Hussain, N., Ali, S.S., Aslam, M. (2022). A Metamaterial Inspired AMC Backed Dual Band Antenna for ISM and RFID Applications. *Sensors* 22, 8065.
22. Arif, A., Zubair, M., Ali, M., Khan, M.U., Mehmood, M.Q. (2019). A Compact, Low-Profile Fractal Antenna for Wearable On-Body WBAN Applications. *IEEE Antennas Wireless Propag Lett* 18(5), 981–985.
23. Choi, D., Shrestha, S., Park, J., Noh, S. (2014). Design and Performance of an Efficient Rectenna Incorporating a Fractal Structure. *Int J Commun Syst* 27, 661–679.

# 3 Thyroid Prediction Using Hybrid CNN and LSTM Model

*Sivakumar Paulraj, Somasundaram Krishnamoorthy, Uma Maheswari, Jayachandran Nagendra Prabhu, Selvaraj Murali Murugan, and Karthikeyan Thiyagarajan*

## 3.1 INTRODUCTION

Thyroid disease is a common endocrine syndrome that affects millions of people worldwide [1]. The thyroid gland, positioned in the front of the neck, plays a major role in regulating metabolism and hormone production. Malfunction of the thyroid gland leads to severe conditions like hypothyroidism, hyperthyroidism, goiter, and thyroid cancer.

Hypothyroidism occurs when the thyroid gland fails to produce an adequate amount of thyroid hormones, resulting in a slowed metabolism and a range of symptoms such as fatigue, weight gain, and depression [2]. Conversely, hyperthyroidism is characterized by the overproduction of thyroid hormones, leading to symptoms such as weight loss, increased heart rate, and anxiety.

Goiter refers to the enlargement of the thyroid gland, often caused by an iodine deficiency or inflammation. While most goiters are benign, some can be a sign of underlying thyroid disorders. The chance of thyroid cancer occurring is very low but thyroid cancer is a potentially serious condition that can develop in the cells of the thyroid gland.

Diagnosing thyroid disease usually contains a combination of clinical evaluation, physical examination, and laboratory tests, including the measurement of thyroid hormone levels and imaging techniques such as ultrasound or scintigraphy [3]. These techniques help healthcare professionals determine the presence and type of thyroid disorder, guiding appropriate treatment decisions.

The accuracy of thyroid disease prediction can be improved by integrating artificial intelligence (AI), such as deep and machine learning models [4]. These techniques have shown hopeful results in automating the detection and classification of thyroid diseases from data sets, permitting faster and more accurate predictions.

DOI: 10.1201/9781003449058-3

### 3.1.1 Convolutional Neural Network (CNN)

CNN architecture is widely employed in data mining tasks due to its ability to extract spatial features and patterns from structured and unstructured datasets. The architecture of CNN consists of an Input Layer, Convolutional Layer (CL), Activation Function, Pooling Layer (PL), Flattening (F), and Fully Connected Layers (FCL). The CNN takes input data in the form of matrices or text. The core component of CNN is the convolutional layer. It consists of multiple filters or kernels that slide over the input data, performing element-wise multiplications and generating feature maps. These filters capture local patterns and detect spatial features within the data.

An activation function is applied to create a non-linearity to the output of the convolutional layer. Common activation functions used in CNN include the Rectified Linear Unit (ReLU), which helps in modeling complex relationships within the data.

Following the 'CL', a 'PL' is typically included. The operations of dimensions reductions and down sampling are carried out in this layer. Max pooling is a common voting approach where the highest value within a predefined pool size is selected, retaining the most salient features. After the 'PL', the feature maps are flattened into a one-dimensional vector. This transformation facilitates further processing by 'FCL'. The flattened features are passed through 'FCL'. These layers consist of neurons that are connected to all neurons in the past layers. FCL's learn high-level representations and capture complex relationships between features.

The final fully connected layer produces the desired output based on the specific task, such as classification labels or predictions. The number of neurons in the output layer depends on the desired output dimensionality. The CNN is trained using a labeled dataset through a process called backpropagation. During training, the model's parameters, including filter weights and biases, are iteratively altered to reduce a defined loss function. This optimization process allows the CNN to learn optimal representations and feature combinations specific to the task at hand.

### 3.1.2 Long Short-Term Memory (LSTM)

LSTM is a modified version of a recurrent network which holds data in a memory unit for learning spatial features. The architecture of the LSTM model is shown in Figure 3.1. The major components of LSTM models are the LSTM cell and gates.

The LSTM model takes input in the form of sequential data, such as time series data or text. The memory cells of the model help capture and retain information over long sequences. Each memory cell consists of three main elements: an input gate (IG), a forget gate (FG), and an output gate (OG). The input gate is responsible for controlling the amount of data to be added into the memory cell. It decides data importance by calculating the sigmoid functions between present and past input data. The forget gate is responsible for deleting unnecessary data to the next state. It decides on deletion by calculating the sigmoid of present and past hidden state values. The functions of gate outputs and LSTM outputs can be seen below:

$$f_t = \sigma(W_{xf}.x_t + .W_{hf}.h_t - 1 + b_f) \tag{3.1}$$

$$i_t = \sigma(W_{xi}.x_t + .W_{hi}.h_t - 1 + b_i) \tag{3.2}$$

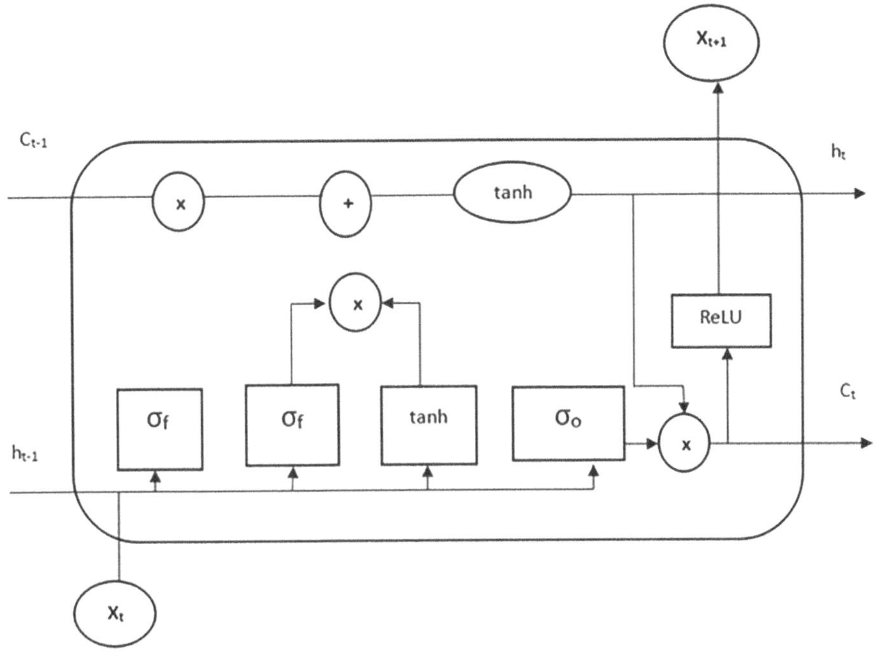


**FIGURE 3.1** Architecture of LSTM model.

$$c\bar{}\_t = \tanh(W\_xc.x\_t + .W\_hc.h\_t \text{ -1 } +b\_c) \tag{3.3}$$

$$c\_t = f\_t*c\_(t\text{-}1)+i\_t*c\bar{}\_t \tag{3.4}$$

$$O\_t = \sigma(W\_xo.x\_t + W\_ho.h\_t \text{ -1 } +b\_o) \tag{3.5}$$

$$h\_t =O\_t*\tanh \tag{3.6}$$

$$y\_t = \sigma(W\_hy.h\_t + b\_y) \tag{3.7}$$

$$\sigma(x)=1/(1+e\text{^}(-x)) \tag{3.8}$$

where f_t, i_t, and O_t represent the FG, IG, and OG functions with weights of W_xf, W_xi, and W_xo, respectively. b represents the bias values of activation functions. The cell state represents the long-term memory of the module. It is updated based on the 'IG' and 'FG' values. The current input, previous hidden state, and the gates' outputs are combined to update the cell state using a 'tanh' activation function. The 'OG' controls the information to be passed from the memory cell to the output. It decides for deletion by calculating the sigmoid of present and past hidden state values. The hidden state is the output of the LSTM cell and represents the short-term memory or the relevant information extracted from the input sequence. It is computed based on the updated cell state and the output gate. The LSTM model is trained using a labeled dataset through backpropagation. The parameters of the LSTM, including the weights and biases, are altered iteratively to reduce a defined loss function. This process allows the LSTM to learn patterns and relationships within the sequential data. By utilizing memory cells and capturing long-term dependencies, LSTM models are particularly effective in tasks involving sequential or time-dependent data.

In this work, a hybrid CNN and LSTM model for thyroid prediction is proposed which combines spatial and temporal information to improve the accuracy for thyroid disease detection. The early detection of thyroid disease supports timely treatments and reduces rates of mortality. This work uses the advantages of DL for early prediction with a smaller number of clinical data.

## 3.2 RELATED WORK

Numerous research groups have conducted significant studies in the field of medical data mining, focusing on various aspects of this domain. In this section, a summary of selected works conducted by researchers in data mining algorithms are provided, highlighting their key findings and contributions.

R. V. Reddy et al. [5] proposed a ML-based thyroid prediction model for higher accuracy. The proposed model includes two steps: Linear Discriminant Analysis (LDA)-based feature extraction and random forest (RF) ML-based classification. The important features from thyroid are extracted using LDA, then, the extracted features are classified by classifier. The accuracy reached by the developed model is 97%.

An ensemble learning model for thyroid prediction was proposed by A. Tyagi et al. [6]. It combines a support vector machine (SVM), RF and naïve Bayes for prediction initially, the features are identified using independent component analysis. Then, ensemble learning with voting is applied for the final classification.

The concept of autoencoder-based feature extraction mechanism was proposed by J. Kim et al. [7]. In an autoencoder, the hidden layer functions as a feature extraction layer, processing the input data into a compressed representation.. The proposed prediction model uses stacking of autoencoders for feature extraction and the final layer is trained to perform the prediction. Compared to other feature learning models, the autoencoder-based model shows higher feature learning capability.

A combined ML and DL-based thyroid prediction model was developed by A. Kumar Pandey et al. [8]. For feature extraction, the Non-Negative Matrix Factorization has been used. The results from different classifiers are used for the final prediction result.

Compared to single models, the accuracy of an ensemble model is higher due to the consideration of outputs from different models or classifiers. In ensemble models, the prediction results of input data are calculated from different models parallelly and then combined by soft voting for final results. This strategy has been applied for thyroid prediction by D. Priyadharsini et al. [9]. The accuracy of the model can be varied based on the adjustments of varying individual model weights.

The performance of the prediction model can be improved by applying optimization algorithms. The optimization genetic algorithm was applied for feature extraction and selection by S. Kurnaz et al. [10] for thyroid disease prediction. Compared to other models, the genetic-based algorithm shows higher accuracy.

K. K. Mahurkar et al. [11] presented a hybrid model for thyroid diagnosis. The hybrid model combines kmeans with a neural network model for classification. The features are identified using kmeans and a neural network is used for final classification. Experiential results on a Kaggle data set shows an accuracy of 97.86% is reached as an average of different cross validation processes.

The concept of rotation transformation was applied in classifiers introduced by Q. Pan et al. [12] for thyroid disease classification. The proposed model involves two steps: Principal Component Analysis for data normalization and pre-processing, and RF for classification. The accuracy of the model was increased by 4.5% due to the integration of rotation transformation.

S. Balasubramanian et al. [13] presented a recurrent neural network-based thyroid disorder prediction model. The recurrent neural network is well suited for handling spatial data of thyroid patients. Three important features were extracted for accurate prediction.

A novel three-stage prediction framework was proposed by M. Karmeni et al. [14] for thyroid disease prediction. It involves pre-processing data imbalance handling and prediction. The data is normalized in pre-processing. To handle data imbalance, data sampling is applied. Finally, the stacked model is used for prediction.

S. Ambesange et al. [15] proposed a pre-processing model for disease prediction. The data outliers and imbalance are handled by sampling techniques. For classification, the refinement model has been used. Also, parameter tuning is used for further accuracy improvement.

The performance of different ML algorithms was analyzed by G. Shukla et al. [16] for disease prediction. Among the different models, a decision tree achieved the highest accuracy and precision rate. They also concluded that the feature selection process shows a major impact on the performance of the classifier model.

R. Zhao et al. [17] introduced a thyroid disease prediction model based on the catboost algorithm. The major advantage of the catboost algorithm is automatic feature scaling and robust overfitting. The encoder types are automatically configured based on the data set nature. The proposed model was evaluated for a data set which contains 673 records. The catboost algorithm reached an accuracy level of 89.98%.

The concept of attention mechanism was proposed Y. An et al. [18] for cardiovascular diseases (CVD) prediction. The DL model is an attention mechanism that improves the feature selection capability of the model for disease prediction. The high-quality feature filtered unwanted features from the data set using attention mechanisms. The results were analyzed for different public data sets.

An AdaBoost and LSTM combined disease severity prediction model was developed by K. Guo et al. [19]. Initially, the features were selected using a clustering process. Then, the combined AdaBoost and LSTM model was applied for feature classification.

A time aware DL model was introduced by Y. An et al. [20] for CVD prediction. The DL model fuses from the prediction results of both CNN and LSTM.

This integration supports considering both temporal and non-temporal features for accurate CVD prediction.

T. Gangavarapu et al. [21] developed a disease risk analysis model using a self-attention mechanism. This strategy was used to tune the network layer parameters for varying data set inputs. Also, the new attribute selection technique was combined for achieving accuracy improvements.

Y. Shen et al. [22] constructed a disease severity classification model that integrates a scoring mechanism and gradient boosting. The gradient boosting is utilized in the classifier for combining the results of different DL models. The scoring system is utilized to optimally select a DL model based on its feature learning capacity. J. W. Phegley et al. [23] developed a risk assessment model for Alzheimer's disease (AD) using a neural network. The autoencoder is processed for feature extraction in clinical data. Then, an electro static neural network is applied for final AD risk classification.

L. Brand et al. [24] presented a LSTM-based clinical disease support system for multiple diseases. The multi regression model was used for feature extraction and classification. Among the existing models, the LSTM model shows higher accuracy in public available data sets. M. Piñol et al. [25] developed a tool to diagnose different diseases for humans. It uses ML and DL models for the assessments. The authors H. Li [26] and G. Yu et al. [27] proposed a DL model for various disease predictions. This model used LSTM models for processing input data and reached a maximum accuracy of 96.87%.

R. Wang et al. [28] proposed a CNN-based COVID-19 disease prediction model. The severity of the patients was computed based on different attributes collected from health care data. The hybrid RF and decision tree model was proposed by S. Mohan et al. [29] for CVD predictions. The maximum accuracy reached by the model was 89.89%.

A fuzzy logic integrated SVM model was proposed by U. Ahmed et al. [30] for diabetic disease prediction. The fuzzy logic processed data sets for feature selection by applying membership rules. Then, SVM was applied for classification. S. M. M. Elkholy et al. [31] presented an improved Deep Belief Network (DBN) to predict chronic kidney disease prediction. Experimental results on the DBN model showed that the model can classify the disease with an accuracy 94.5% and an F-score rate of 90.3% compared with previous ones. A generative adversarial network (GAN) model-based disease prediction model was presented by X. Jiang et al. [32]. The GAN model is combined with autoencoders for accurate disease prediction.

The challenges physicians face in these areas are multifaceted. Accessing and integrating diverse data sources, such as clinical parameters, imaging data, genetic profiles, and treatment records, can be time-consuming and complex. Traditional relational databases often pose difficulties in retrieving comprehensive diagnostic summaries and assessing disease severities due to their relational nature and complex data structures. Similarly, identifying and linking adverse effects to specific treatments or comorbidity conditions can be challenging, as relevant information is scattered across various database tables and lacks standardized terminology.

## 3.3 PROTOTYPE ARCHITECTURE DEVELOPMENT AND FUNCTIONALITY

The proposed prediction model consists of two major blocks: a CNN module for feature extraction and an LSTM for final classification as shown in Figure 3.2. The CNN component extracts relevant features from the clinical data set, capturing spatial information. The extracted features are then fed into the LSTM model, which learns the temporal dependencies and patterns within the sequence of data.

The CNN component starts with a 1D convolutional layer (Conv1D) that applies multiple filters to the input sequence. This layer efficiently identifies local patterns and features within the data. Subsequently, a max pooling layer (MaxPooling1D) reduces the spatial dimensions of the feature maps, capturing the relevant features for thyroid prediction. To avoid overfitting, a 'DL' is introduced, randomly setting a fraction of input units to zero during training. Finally, a 'FL' transforms the output into a one-dimensional vector, ready for further processing.

The LSTM component is designed to observe the temporal dependencies of thyroid data. The LSTM processes this data with memory cells. This layer learns the patterns over time, allowing the model to understand the thyroid data which affects majorly for prediction. To regularize the LSTM layer and further prevent overfitting, a dropout layer is included.

The 'OL' of the model is a dense layer, which produces the final prediction based on the learned features from the CNN and LSTM components. In this work, three stages of thyroid disease are classified; therefore, the number of neurons in the output layer (OL) is set to three.. By combining these two components, the model can effectively learn both spatial and temporal data from thyroid clinical data, leading to improved accuracy in thyroid prediction.

### 3.3.1 Hyperparameter Tuning

In the hybrid CNN and LSTM model, there are many hyperparameters that need to be tuned for optimal prediction results. These hyperparameters contribute a major role in its accuracy. Tuning these hyperparameters is necessary to tune the right balance between model complexity and generalization.

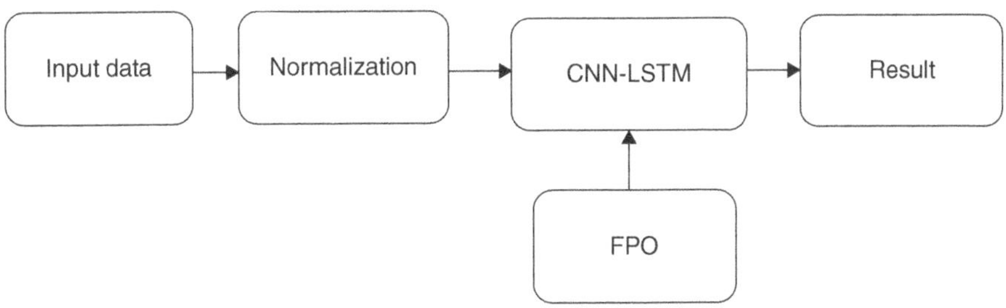


**FIGURE 3.2** Proposed architecture.

One important hyperparameter is the number of CNN layers, which determines the depth of the CNN component in the model. Increasing the number of CNN layers allows for capturing more complex spatial features. However, finding the optimal balance is crucial to prevent overfitting and to ensure that the model can generalize well for unseen data.

Similarly, the number of LSTM layers is a critical hyperparameter that affects the depth of the LSTM component. Adding more LSTM layers enables the model to capture intricate temporal dependencies within the data. However, the number of layers should be chosen carefully, as increasing complexity may require more data and computational resources.

The filter size and stride hyperparameters in the CNN component play a major role in determining the receptive field of the filters and the step size when moving them across the input data. Proper tuning of these hyperparameters is essential to ensure that the model can capture spatial patterns at different scales effectively.

Another vital hyperparameter is the dropout rate, which determines the fraction of neurons that are randomly dropped out during training. By preventing overfitting, dropout regularization helps the model generalize better to unseen data. Careful tuning of the dropout rate is necessary to find the right balance between model complexity and generalization performance.

The learning rate hyperparameter controls the step size at which the model's parameters are updated during training. It plays a critical role in the training dynamics and the model's ability to converge to an optimal solution. Finding an appropriate learning rate is crucial to ensure efficient training and avoid getting stuck in sub-optimal solutions or diverging.

Other hyperparameters, such as batch size, which determines the number of samples processed before updating the model's parameters, and the number of epochs, which defines how many times the model goes through the entire training dataset, also require careful tuning. These hyperparameters influence training dynamics, memory requirements, and generalization capabilities. In this work, an optimization algorithm, the Flower Pollination Optimization Algorithm (FPOA), is used for hyperparameter tuning.

### 3.3.2 Flower Pollination Optimization Algorithm (FPOA)

FFPOA is a nature-inspired optimization algorithm that emulates the pollination behavior of flowers. It uses the transfer of pollen grains to achieve cross-pollination and genetic diversity. The algorithm operates by iteratively updating candidate solutions using the following equations:

Flower Pollination Equation:

$$X(t+1) = X(t) + beta * (X(t) - X(poll)) \tag{3.9}$$

In Equation (3.9), X(t) represents the current candidate solution, X(t+1) is the updated solution, X(poll) is a randomly selected solution from the population, and beta is a randomization parameter.

Fitness Function Evaluation:

$$F(X(t+1)) \quad (3.10)$$

Equation (3.10) evaluates the fitness of the updated solution X(t+1) using a predefined fitness function F. The fitness function depends on the specific optimization problem being solved.

Flower Communication and Pollen Dispersal:

$$X(t+1) = X(t+1) + sigma * L * (X(bettersol) - X(worstsol)) \quad (3.11)$$

Equation (3.11) incorporates flower communication and pollen dispersal. Here, X(bettersol) represents the best solution found so far, X(worstsol) is the worst solution, sigma is a randomization parameter, and L is the levy flight operator used to explore the search space.

By iteratively applying Equations (3.9) to (3.11), the FPOA algorithm discovers the solution space, aiming to converge towards the global optimum. The algorithm combines randomization, local search, and the concept of flower pollination to efficiently find optimal solutions for various optimization problems. The pseudo code for proposed parameter tuning is given below

**Initialize** population of candidate solutions
**Define** the fitness function to evaluate the performance of the CNN-LSTM model
**Set** maximum number of iterations
**Set** the number of flowers in the population
**Set** the number of flowers for pollen dispersal
**Set** the randomization parameter (beta) and the levy flight parameter (sigma)
**Initialize** the best solution found so far (best_sol)
**Initialize** the worst solution (worst_sol)
**Repeat** for each iteration until convergence or maximum iterations reached:
    **Evaluate** fitness for each candidate solution in the population
    **Update** best_sol and worst_sol based on the fitness values
    **For** each candidate solution X:
        **Select** a random solution from the population (poll)
        **Generate** a new solution using Equation (3.10): X_new = X + beta * (X - poll)
        **Evaluate** the fitness of X_new using the fitness function
        Perform flower communication and pollen dispersal using Equation (3.11):
        X_new = X_new + sigma * levy_flight_operator * (best_sol - worst_sol)
        **Replace** X with X_new if it has better fitness than X
**Return** the best solution found (best_sol)

The algorithm initializes a population of candidate solutions representing different configurations of the CNN-LSTM architecture. The fitness function assesses the performance of each candidate's outcomes. The algorithm iteratively updates the solutions based on the FPOA equations, including randomization, flower communication, and pollen dispersal. At each iteration, the best and worst solutions are updated based on their fitness values. The algorithm continues until convergence is reached, returning the best solution found.

### 3.3.3 Parameter Tuning Using Optimizer

The Coot optimization algorithm is a new meta-heuristic method inspired by the behavior of a swarm of birds called Coots. This algorithm is designed to solve complex engineering problems by searching for the optimal solution in the search space which applies exploration and exploitation stages. The Coot algorithm consists of four phases to reach best solution:

### 3.3.4 Random Movement

During the first phase, the movement of the swarm of coots is irregular. The stages involve random perturbations to explore the solution space in a broad and diverse manner. To avoid reaching local minima, this stage explores different regions of the search space. The random movement is expressed as follows:

$$P=r*(1,d)*(ul-ll)+ll \tag{3.12}$$

where, r is the random number and ul and ll are the upper and lower limits of optimization, respectively.

### 3.3.5 Chain Movement

Chain movement is the second stage of the optimization process to find the best solution. The movements of the coots become regular, resembling a chain-like formation. Each coot travels behind its front coot, creating a sequential alignment. This chain movement is helpful for exploration and exploitation of hopeful areas in the search space. Based on the chain movement, the algorithm escaped from local minima. The update position in this phase is expressed as follows:

$$P=0.5*(P(i-1)+P(i)) \tag{3.13}$$

### 3.3.6 Adjusting the Position Based on the Group Leaders

In this phase, the coots adjust their positions based on the information provided by the group leaders. The group leaders are those coots that have found better solutions or more promising areas in the search space. The other coots align their movements based on the positions of these leaders, allowing them to benefit from the information gathered by the successful coots. The update position based on leader position (LP) in this phase is expressed as follows:

$$P=LP(k)+2randcos(2.14)*LP) \tag{3.14}$$

### 3.3.7 Leading the Group by the Leaders

The final phase involves the leaders leading the entire swarm towards the optimal area in the search space. The leaders' movements are influential in guiding the swarm towards better solutions. As the leaders adjust their positions based on their search experiences, the swarm converges towards better solutions over time.

The Coot optimization algorithm imitates the collective behavior of a swarm of birds, employing random exploration, chain-like movement, group leader influence, and convergence towards optimal areas. By combining these phases, the algorithm efficiently explores the search space and converges towards high-quality solutions for complex engineering problems.

### 3.3.8 Hyperparameter Tuning Using Cook

The hyperparameters of the CNN model include Kernel Size, Stride, Padding, Number of Filters, and Activation Function and Pooling, Pooling layers, and average-pooling layers. The hyperparameters of the LSTM model include Number of LSTM Units, Dropout Rate, Recurrent Dropout Rate, and Activation Function

These hyperparameters are tuned to find the optimal combination that yields the best performance of the CNN-LSTM model on thyroid prediction. Hyperparameter tuning is essential to avoid overfitting or underfitting the model, achieve better generalization, and improve overall model performance. In this work, the hyperparameters are tuned using the cook optimizer. The pseudocode for parameter tuning using the cook optimizer is given below:

```
def coot_optimization(num_coots, max_generations, ul, ll):
        # Initialize the swarm of coots with random positions
        swarm = initialize_swarm(num_coots, ul, ll)
           for generation in range(max_generations):
           for coot in swarm:
              # Phase 1: Random Movement
              P_new = random_movement(coot.position, ul, ll)
                        # Phase 2: Chain Movement
              P_new = chain_movement(coot.position, swarm)
                        # Phase 3: Adjusting Position Based on Group Leaders
              P_new = leader_adjustment(coot.position, best_leader_position(swarm))
     # Evaluate the hybrid CNN-LSTM model using the hyperparameters
     P_new coot.fitness = evaluate_model(P_new)
                          # Update the position of the coot if the new position is better
              if coot.fitness < coot.best_fitness:
                 coot.best_position = P_new
                 coot.best_fitness = coot.fitness
     # Phase 4: Leading the Group by the Leaders Towards the Optimal Area
     (Leader Movement)
          update_leader_positions(swarm)
          # Return the best hyperparameter set found in the swarm
       return best_coot_position(swarm)
```

## 3.4 RESULTS AND DISCUSSION

The data set is collected from Kaggle web site (www.kaggle.com/code/yasserhessein/thyroid-disease-detection-using-deep-learning/notebook). The data set includes different attributes for thyroid prediction. It includes the fields of age, gender, and medication history, including whether they are on thyroxine or antithyroid medication. It also includes medicines taken during previous treatments. The different attributes may cause different impacts on prediction accuracy. The data set also includes the levels of Thyroid-Stimulating Hormone (TSH), Triiodothyronine (T3), Total Thyroxine (TT4), Thyroxine Uptake (T4U), Free Thyroxine Index (FTI), and Thyroxine-Binding Globulin (TBG). The data set also includes information about whether these measurements were taken.

The performance of the proposed model is analyzed in terms of Precision, Recall, Accuracy, F1 score, Root Mean Squared Error (RMSE), and Mean Absolute Error (MAE). This parameter can be obtained by substituting true positives (TP), false positives (FP), false negatives (FN), and true negatives (TN) of the results.

$$\text{Precision (\%)} = (TP / (TP + FP)) * 100 \tag{3.15}$$

$$\text{Recall (\%)} = (TP / (TP + FN)) * 100 \tag{3.16}$$

$$\text{Accuracy (\%)} = ((TP + TN) / (TP + TN + FP + FN)) * 100 \tag{3.17}$$

$$\text{F1 score (\%)} = (2 * \text{Precision} * \text{Recall}) / (\text{Precision} + \text{Recall}) * 100 \tag{3.18}$$

$$\text{RMSE} = \text{sqrt}((1/N) * \text{sum}((\text{predicted - actual})\hat{}2)) \tag{3.19}$$

$$\text{MAE} = (1/N) * \text{sum}(\text{abs}(\text{predicted - actual}) \tag{3.20}$$

The model takes an input and produces an output of shape (None, 1), indicating a single value prediction. The first layer is a dense layer with 256 neurons. Each neuron in this layer is connected to every neuron in the previous layer. The output shape of this layer is (None, 256). It has a total of 7,424 trainable parameters, which are modified during the training.

Following the 'CL', a 'DL' is applied. It randomly sets a fraction of input units to 0 during training to avoid overfitting. The output shape remains the same as the previous layer (None, 256), and this layer does not have any trainable parameters. The attributes of dataset values are visualized as shown in Figure 3.3,

The evaluation results of proposed model are shown in Figure 3.4. It reveals a continued positive trend in the model's performance. The training loss decreases to 0.0261, indicating the model's increasing accuracy in predicting outcomes on the training data. The accuracy results of the proposed model are given in Figure 3.5.

The performance of the proposed model is given in Table 3.1. The CNN-LSTM model exhibits exceptional performance across multiple evaluation measures, proving its effectiveness for prediction. With a precision of 98.43%, the CNN-LSTM model demonstrates a high level of accuracy in correctly identifying positive predictions.

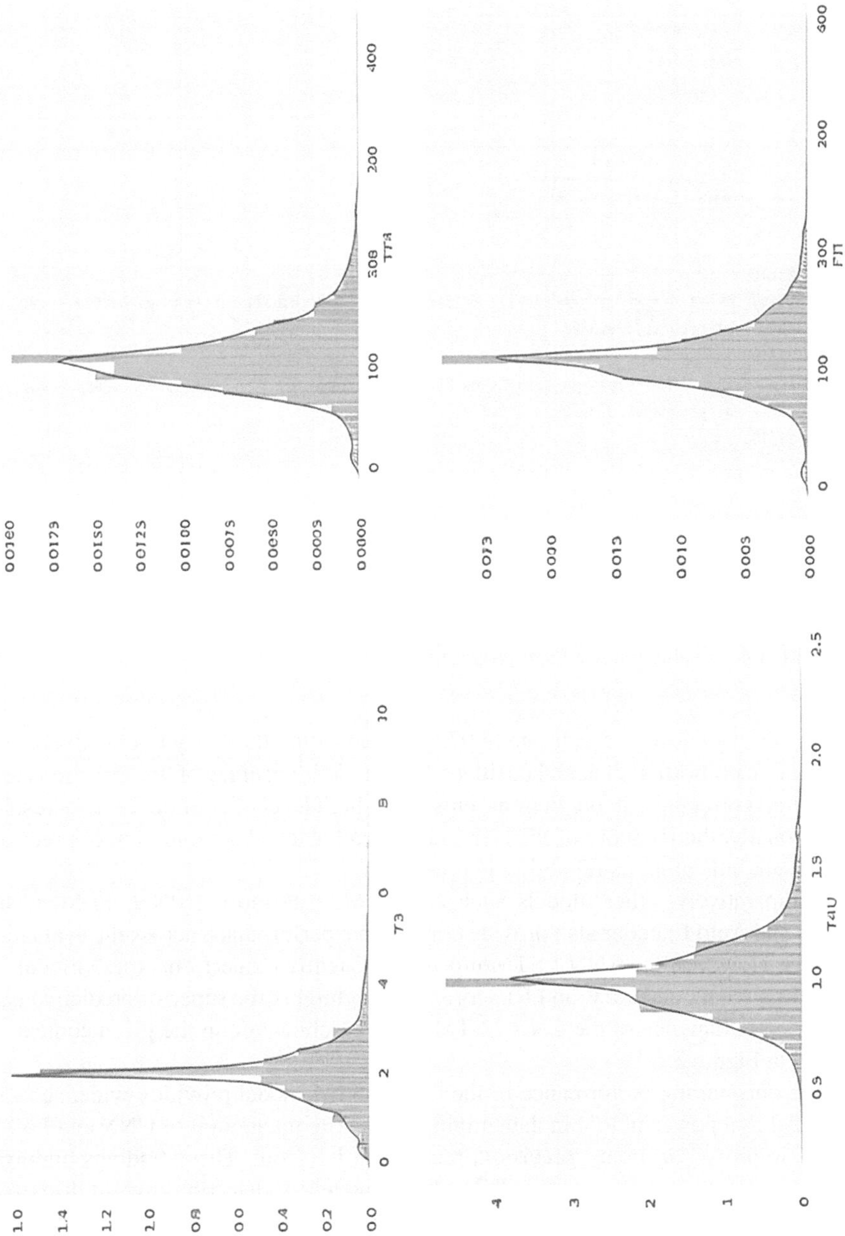

**FIGURE 3.3** Visualization of attributes.

```
Layer (type)                 Output Shape              Param #
================================================================
dense (Dense)                (None, 256)               7424
________________________________________________________________
dropout (Dropout)            (None, 256)               0
________________________________________________________________
dense_1 (Dense)              (None, 128)               32800
________________________________________________________________
dropout_1 (Dropout)          (None, 128)               0
________________________________________________________________
dense_2 (Dense)              (None, 63)                8127
________________________________________________________________
dropout_2 (Dropout)          (None, 63)                0
________________________________________________________________
dense_3 (Dense)              (None, 1)                 64
================================================================
Total params: 48,511
Trainable params: 48,511
Non-trainable params: 0
________________________________________________________________

Epoch 24/100
40/40 [==============================] - 0s 3ms/step - loss: 0.0371 - accuracy: 0.9839 - val_los
s: 0.0405 - val_accuracy: 0.9823
Epoch 25/100
40/40 [==============================] - 0s 3ms/step - loss: 0.0322 - accuracy: 0.9882 - val_los
s: 0.0257 - val_accuracy: 0.9929
Epoch 26/100
40/40 [==============================] - 0s 3ms/step - loss: 0.0331 - accuracy: 0.9882 - val_los
s: 0.0196 - val_accuracy: 0.9894
Epoch 27/100
40/40 [==============================] - 0s 3ms/step - loss: 0.0261 - accuracy: 0.9886 - val_los
s: 0.0172 - val_accuracy: 0.9894
Epoch 28/100
```

**FIGURE 3.4** Evaluation results of proposed model.

Moreover, it achieves a recall rate of 97.54%, indicating its ability to effectively capture a large proportion of actual positives. The model's accuracy of 96.77% showcases its overall correctness in predictions, ensuring a high level of confidence in its results. Additionally, the F1 score of 97.45% indicates a balanced combination of precision and recall, indicating its reliability in prediction.

Comparatively, other models such as LSTM, AdaBoost, BPNN, ELM, CNN, SVM, and Auto Encoder also provide competitive performance across the evaluation metrics. However, the CNN-LSTM model consistently outperforms these models in precision, recall, accuracy, and F1 score. This highlights the superior predictive capability and efficiency of the CNN-LSTM hybrid architecture in the given context, as shown in Figure 3.6.

The outstanding performance of the CNN-LSTM model provides evidence of its potential as a powerful tool in data mining tasks. The integration of CNN and LSTM shows improved accuracy, precision, recall, and F1 score. These findings highlight the significance of the proposed CNN-LSTM model for detecting thyroid disease in different environments.

The CNN-LSTM model demonstrated outstanding performance, achieving a precision of 98.43%. When compared to the LSTM model, the CNN-LSTM exhibited a considerable increment of approximately 1.88%. Similarly, in contrast to the

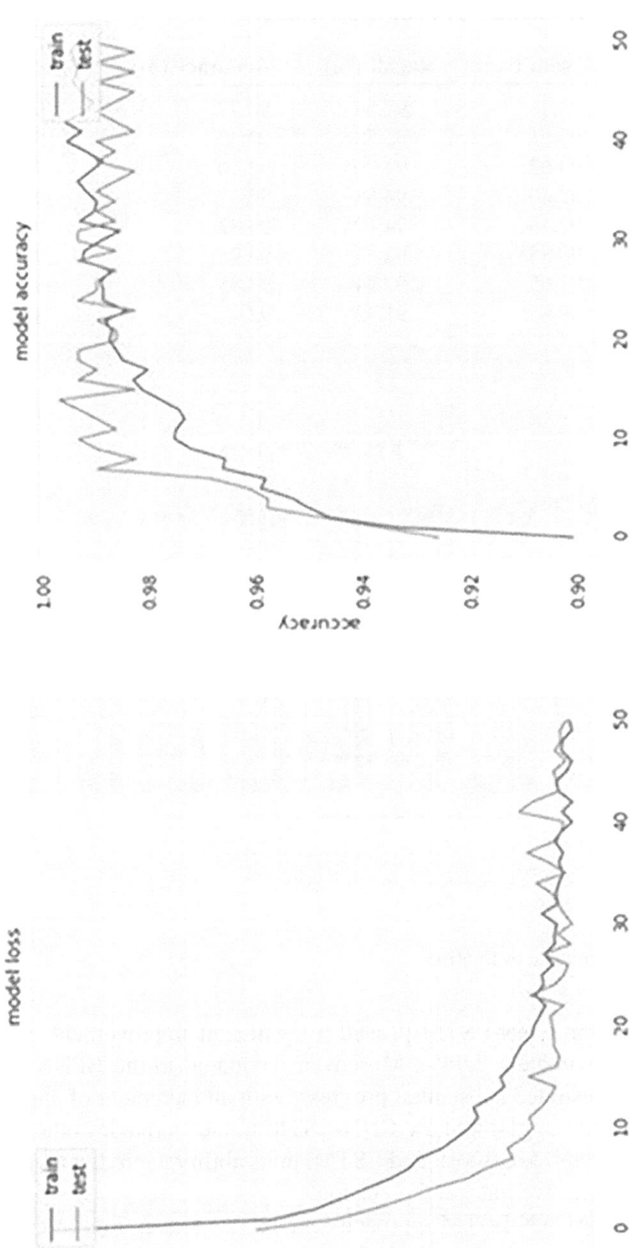


**FIGURE 3.5** Accuracy results.

**TABLE 3.1**
**Performance Metrics Result of Proposed Model**

| Techniques | Precision (%) | Recall (%) | Accuracy (%) | $F_1$ score (%) |
|---|---|---|---|---|
| CNN-LSTM | 98.43 | 97.54 | 96.77 | 97.45 |
| LSTM | 96.61 | 95.58 | 94.49 | 93.74 |
| AdaBoost | 95.62 | 94.26 | 94.10 | 92.33 |
| BPNN | 92.40 | 94.58 | 94 | 91.24 |
| ELM | 92.48 | 94.12 | 94.32 | 91.21 |
| CNN | 90.85 | 92.55 | 93.2 | 90.11 |
| SVM | 91.65 | 92.44 | 92.85 | 89.23 |
| Auto Encoder | 89.66 | 91.42 | 92 | 88.52 |

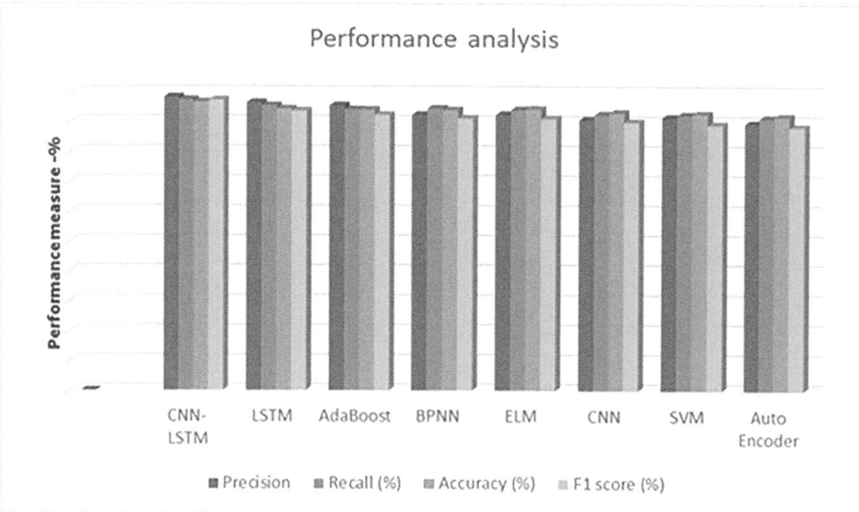


**FIGURE 3.6** Performance evaluation.

AdaBoost model, the CNN-LSTM proved a significant improvement, boasting an increment of approximately 2.94%. Moreover, compared to the BPNN model, the CNN-LSTM demonstrated substantial progress, with an increment of approximately 6.03%. These results suggest that the CNN-LSTM model surpasses other traditional models, such as BPNN, AdaBoost, and LSTM, in its ability to predict thyroid-related outcomes with greater accuracy and precision.

For recall rate, the CNN-LSTM approach demonstrated exceptional recall performance, achieving an impressive recall of 97.54%. A comparative analysis revealed that the CNN-LSTM model outperformed other techniques significantly. When compared to the LSTM model, the CNN-LSTM provided an increment of approximately 2.05% in recall accuracy. Similarly, compared to the AdaBoost, BPNN, and ELM models, the CNN-LSTM displayed substantial increments of approximately 3.47%, 3.14%, and 3.63%, respectively. Furthermore, the CNN-LSTM model exhibited remarkable superiority over traditional models like CNN and SVM, with increments of approximately 5.38% and 5.49%, respectively. Even when pitted against the Auto Encoder model, the CNN-LSTM proved to be the superior choice, with an increment of approximately 6.12%. These results highlight the CNN-LSTM model's remarkable capability to predict thyroid-related outcomes with higher recall percentages, making it a promising candidate for accurate and reliable thyroid prediction tasks.

For accuracy analysis, the CNN-LSTM model proved to be a standout performer, attaining an impressive accuracy of 96.77%. When compared to other models, the CNN-LSTM consistently provided significant improvements. Compared to the LSTM model, the CNN-LSTM exhibited a substantial increment of approximately 2.41% in accuracy. Similarly, in comparison to the AdaBoost, BPNN, and ELM models, the CNN-LSTM displayed noteworthy increments of approximately 2.84%, 2.95%, and 2.60%, respectively. Furthermore, the CNN-LSTM model demonstrated notable superiority over conventional models like CNN and SVM, with increments of approximately 3.82% and 4.14%, respectively. Even when compared to the Auto Encoder model, the CNN-LSTM exhibited remarkable progress, with an increment of approximately 4.77%. These findings underscore the CNN-LSTM model's exceptional potential to predict thyroid-related outcomes with heightened accuracy, making it a highly promising choice for reliable and precise thyroid prediction tasks.

For F1 score analysis, when compared to other models, the CNN-LSTM consistently demonstrated substantial improvements. In contrast to the LSTM model, the CNN-LSTM showcased a remarkable increment of approximately 3.96% in F1 score accuracy. Similarly, when compared to the AdaBoost, BPNN, and ELM models, the CNN-LSTM displayed significant increments of approximately 5.54%, 6.79%, and 6.89%, respectively. Moreover, the CNN-LSTM model exhibited noteworthy superiority over traditional models like CNN and SVM, with increments of approximately 8.12% and 9.16%, respectively. Even when compared to the Auto Encoder model, the CNN-LSTM exhibited remarkable progress, with an increment of approximately 10.06%. These findings underscore the CNN-LSTM model's exceptional potential to predict thyroid-related outcomes with heightened F1 score accuracy, positioning it as a highly promising and reliable choice for thyroid prediction tasks.

Comparing the CNN-LSTM model with other models based on the provided RMSE and MAE metrics shows good results for performance, as shown in Table 3.2.

**TABLE 3.2**
**Error Metrics Result of Proposed Model**

| Techniques | RMSE | MAE |
|---|---|---|
| CNN-LSTM | 1.226 | 1.745 |
| LSTM | 3.568 | 3.254 |
| AdaBoost | 3.804 | 3.870 |
| BPNN | 4.158 | 4.961 |
| ELM | 4.043 | 4.860 |
| CNN | 5.175 | 5.978 |
| SVM | 5.458 | 6.265 |
| Auto Encoder | 5.956 | 7.23 |

The CNN-LSTM model stands out with significantly lower RMSE and MAE values, representing its superior accuracy in thyroid prediction of the target variable compared to the other models.

With an RMSE of 1.226 and MAE of 1.745, the CNN-LSTM model proves its ability to minimize the average squared differences between predicted and actual values, resulting in more precise predictions overall. These low error values reflect the model's ability to capture and generalize complex patterns of patient data, leading to highly accurate thyroid disease predictions.

In contrast, the other models such as LSTM, AdaBoost, BPNN, ELM, CNN, SVM, and Auto Encoder exhibit higher RMSE and MAE values, indicating relatively higher prediction errors. This suggests that the proposed model is most suitable for predicting thyroid disease prediction, as shown in Figure 3.7.

The CNN-LSTM model emerged as a clear standout, boasting remarkably low values for both RMSE (1.226) and MAE (1.745). Compared to other models, the CNN-LSTM provided significant reductions in both RMSE and MAE, signifying its superior predictive capabilities. When compared to the LSTM model, the CNN-LSTM achieved an impressive decrement of approximately 65.51% in RMSE and 46.41% in MAE. Similarly, compared to the AdaBoost model, the CNN-LSTM confirmed substantial decrements of approximately 67.74% in RMSE and 55.06% in MAE. Also, the CNN-LSTM model showed significant reductions when compared to the BPNN, ELM, CNN, SVM, and Auto Encoder models, with decrement percentages of approximately 70.41%, 69.54%, 76.28%, 79.21%, and 79.41% in RMSE, respectively, and approximately 64.26%, 64.56%, 67.45%, 72.50%, and 73.60% in MAE, respectively. These findings clearly show the CNN-LSTM model's superior performance and accuracy, making it an exceptional choice for precise and reliable thyroid prediction tasks.

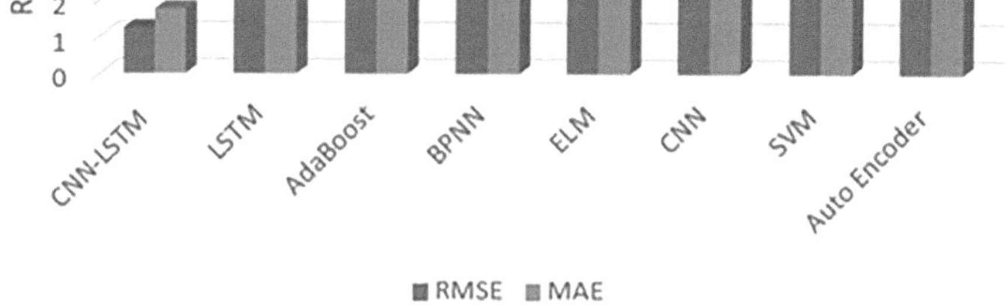


**FIGURE 3.7** Error rate analysis.

## 3.5 CONCLUSION

This work has introduced a hybrid model that combines CNN and LSTM to enhance the accuracy and reliability of thyroid prediction. By integrating the CNN for feature extraction and the LSTM for sequence modeling, the proposed model effectively uses both spatial and temporal information for improved prediction performance.

Comparatively, other models such as LSTM, AdaBoost, BPNN, ELM, CNN, SVM, and Autoencoder also demonstrated competitive performance across the evaluation metrics.

The model's ability to effectively capture meaningful spatial features and temporal patterns contributes to its enhanced performance in thyroid disease detection.

## REFERENCES

1. M. E. Beynon and K. Pinneri, "An Overview of the Thyroid Gland and Thyroid-related Deaths for the Forensic Pathologist," in *Academic Forensic Pathology,* vol. 6, no. 2, pp. 217–236, 2016, DOI: 10.23907/2016.024.
2. K. Paczkowska, A. Otlewska, O. Loska, K. Kolačkov, M. Bolanowski and J. Daroszewski, "Laboratory Interference in the Thyroid Function Test," in *Endokrynologia Polska,* vol. 71, no. 6, pp. 551–560, 2020, DOI: 10.5603/EP.a2020.0079.
3. Q. T. Nguyen, E. J. Lee, M. G. Huang, Y. I. Park, A. Khullar and R. A. Plodkowski, "Diagnosis and Treatment of Patients with Thyroid Cancer," in *American Health & Drug Benefits,* vol. 8, no. 1, pp. 30–40, 2015.
4. L. Ozyilmaz and T. Yildirim, "Diagnosis of Thyroid Disease Using Artificial Neural Network Methods," Proceedings of the 9th International Conference on Neural Information Processing, 2002. ICONIP'02, vol. 4. IEEE, Piscataway, 2002, pp. 2033–2036.
5. R. V. Reddy, G. S. Monisha, A. M. Ali, P. Y. Devi, M. V. Madhusudhan and Y. Sucharitha, "Empirical Method for Thyroid Disease Prediction Using a Deep Learning Techniques," 2023 IEEE 8th International Conference for Convergence in Technology (I2CT), Lonavla, India, 2023, pp. 1–5, DOI: 10.1109/I2CT57861.2023.10126291.
6. A. Tyagi, R. Mehra and A. Saxena, "Interactive Thyroid Disease Prediction System Using Machine Learning Technique," 2018 Fifth International Conference on Parallel, Distributed and Grid Computing (PDGC), Solan, India, 2018, pp. 689–693, DOI: 10.1109/PDGC.2018.8745910.
7. J. Kim and H. Shin, "Prediction of Recurrence Probability of Thyroid Cancer Patients using Similarity Loss-based Multi-modal Autoencoder," 2023 IEEE International Conference on Big Data and Smart Computing (BigComp), Jeju, Republic of Korea, 2023, pp. 358–360, DOI: 10.1109/BigComp57234.2023.00082.
8. A. Kumar Pandey and A. Barve, "Using Deep Neural Network to Detect Thyroid Cancer," 2022 11th International Conference on System Modeling & Advancement in Research Trends (SMART), Moradabad, India, 2022, pp. 1347–1351, DOI: 10.1109/SMART55829.2022.10047782.
9. D. Priyadharsini and S. Sasikala, "Efficient Thyroid Disease Prediction using Features Selection and Meta-Classifiers," 2022 6th International Conference on Computing Methodologies and Communication (ICCMC), Erode, India, 2022, pp. 1236–1243, DOI: 10.1109/ICCMC53470.2022.9753986.

10. S. Kurnaz, M. S. Mohammed and S. J. Mohammed, "A High Efficiency Thyroid Disorders Prediction System with Non-Dominated Sorting Genetic Algorithm NSGA-II as a Feature Selection Algorithm," 2020 International Conference for Emerging Technology (INCET), Belgaum, India, 2020, pp. 1–6, DOI: 10.1109/INCET49848.2020.9154189.
11. K. K. Mahurkar and D. P. Gaikwad, "Normalization Using Improvised K-Means Applied in Diagnosing Thyroid Disease with ANN," 2017 International Conference on Trends in Electronics and Informatics (ICEI), Tirunelveli, India, 2017, pp. 579–583, DOI: 10.1109/ICOEI.2017.8300768.
12. Q. Pan, Y. Zhang, M. Zuo, L. Xiang and D. Chen, "Improved Ensemble Classification Method of Thyroid Disease Based on Random Forest," 2016 8th International Conference on Information Technology in Medicine and Education (ITME), Fuzhou, China, 2016, pp. 567–571, DOI: 10.1109/ITME.2016.0134.
13. S. Balasubramanian, V. Srinivasan and A. Thomo, "Identifying Important Features for Clinical Diagnosis of Thyroid Disorder," 2022 IEEE/ACM International Conference on Advances in Social Networks Analysis and Mining (ASONAM), Istanbul, Turkey, 2022, pp. 363–369, DOI: 10.1109/ASONAM55673.2022.10068712.
14. M. Karmeni, E. B. Abdallah, K. Boukadi and M. Abed, "Towards An Accurate Stacked Ensemble Learning Model for Thyroid Earlier Detection," 2022 IEEE/ACS 19th International Conference on Computer Systems and Applications (AICCSA), Abu Dhabi, United Arab Emirates, 2022, pp. 1–8, DOI: 10.1109/AICCSA56895.2022.10017629.
15. S. Ambesange, A. Vijayalaxmi,, R. Uppin, S. Patil and V. Patil, "Optimizing Liver Disease Prediction with Random Forest by Various Data Balancing Techniques," 2020 IEEE International Conference on Cloud Computing in Emerging Markets (CCEM), Bengaluru, India, 2020, pp. 98–102, DOI: 10.1109/CCEM50674.2020.00030.
16. G. Shukla, G. Dhuriya, S. K. Pillai and A. Saini, "Chronic Kidney Disease Prediction Using Machine Learning Algorithms and the Important Attributes for the Detection," 2023 IEEE IAS Global Conference on Emerging Technologies (GlobConET), London, United Kingdom, 2023, pp. 1–4, DOI: 10.1109/GlobConET56651.2023.10149900.
17. R. Zhao, X. Wen, H. Pang and Z. Ma, "Liver Disease Prediction Using W-LR-XGB Algorithm," 2021 International Conference on Computer, Blockchain and Financial Development (CBFD), Nanjing, China, 2021, pp. 245–248, DOI: 10.1109/CBFD52659.2021.00055.
18. Y. An, N. Huang, X. Chen, F. Wu and J. Wang, "High-Risk Prediction of Cardiovascular Diseases via Attention-Based Deep Neural Networks," in *IEEE/ACM Transactions on Computational Biology and Bioinformatics*, vol. 18, no. 3, pp. 1093–1105, 1 May-June 2021, DOI: 10.1109/TCBB.2019.2935059.
19. K. Guo et al., "Traffic Data-Empowered XGBoost-LSTM Framework for Infectious Disease Prediction," in *IEEE Transactions on Intelligent Transportation Systems*, vol. 25, pp. 774–785, 2022, DOI: 10.1109/TITS.2022.3172206.
20. Y. An, K. Tang and J. Wang, "Time-Aware Multi-Type Data Fusion Representation Learning Framework for Risk Prediction of Cardiovascular Diseases," in *IEEE/ACM Transactions on Computational Biology and Bioinformatics*, vol. 19, no. 6, pp. 3725–3734, 1 Nov.–Dec. 2022, DOI: 10.1109/TCBB.2021.3118418.
21. T. Gangavarapu, G. S. Krishnan, S. Kamath and J. Jeganathan, "FarSight: Long-Term Disease Prediction Using Unstructured Clinical Nursing Notes," in *IEEE Transactions on Emerging Topics in Computing*, vol. 9, no. 3, pp. 1151–1169, 1 July–Sept. 2021, DOI: 10.1109/TETC.2020.2975251.

22. Y. Shen, J. Zhu, Z. Deng, W. Lu and H. Wang, "EnsDeepDP: An Ensemble Deep Learning Approach for Disease Prediction Through Metagenomics," in *IEEE/ACM Transactions on Computational Biology and Bioinformatics*, vol. 20, no. 2, pp. 986–998, 1 March–April 2023, DOI: 10.1109/TCBB.2022.3201295.
23. J. W. Phegley, K. Perkins, L. Gupta and L. F. Hughes, "Multicategory Prediction of Multifactorial Diseases Through Risk Factor Fusion and Rank-sum Selection," in *IEEE Transactions on Systems, Man, and Cybernetics – Part A: Systems and Humans*, vol. 35, no. 5, pp. 718–726, Sept. 2005, DOI: 10.1109/TSMCA.2005.843390.
24. L. Brand, K. Nichols, H. Wang, L. Shen and H. Huang, "Joint Multi-Modal Longitudinal Regression and Classification for Alzheimer's Disease Prediction," in *IEEE Transactions on Medical Imaging*, vol. 39, no. 6, pp. 1845–1855, June 2020, DOI: 10.1109/TMI.2019.2958943.
25. M. Piñol, R. Alves, I. Teixidó, J. Mateo, F. Solsona and E. Vilaprinyó, "Rare Disease Discovery: An Optimized Disease Ranking System," in *IEEE Transactions on Industrial Informatics*, vol. 13, no. 3, pp. 1184–1192, June 2017, DOI: 10.1109/TII.2017.2686380.
26. H. Li, X. Li, M. Ramanathan and A. Zhang, "Prediction and Informative Risk Factor Selection of Bone Diseases," in *IEEE/ACM Transactions on Computational Biology and Bioinformatics*, vol. 12, no. 1, pp. 79–91, 1 Jan.–Feb. 2015, DOI: 10.1109/TCBB.2014.2330579.
27. G. Yu, Y. Yang, Y. Yan, M. Guo, X. Zhang and J. Wang, "DeepIDA: Predicting Isoform-Disease Associations by Data Fusion and Deep Neural Networks," in *IEEE/ACM Transactions on Computational Biology and Bioinformatics*, vol. 19, no. 4, pp. 2166–2176, 1 July–Aug. 2022, DOI: 10.1109/TCBB.2021.3058801.
28. R. Wang, C. Ji, Z. Jiang, Y. Wu, L. Yin and Y. Li, "A Short-Term Prediction Model at the Early Stage of the COVID-19 Pandemic Based on Multisource Urban Data," in *IEEE Transactions on Computational Social Systems*, vol. 8, no. 4, pp. 938–945, Aug. 2021, DOI: 10.1109/TCSS.2021.3060952.
29. S. Mohan, C. Thirumalai and G. Srivastava, "Effective Heart Disease Prediction Using Hybrid Machine Learning Techniques," in *IEEE Access*, vol. 7, pp. 81542–81554, 2019, DOI: 10.1109/ACCESS.2019.2923707.
30. U. Ahmed et al., "Prediction of Diabetes Empowered with Fused Machine Learning," in *IEEE Access*, vol. 10, pp. 8529–8538, 2022, DOI: 10.1109/ACCESS.2022.3142097.
31. S. M. M. Elkholy, A. Rezk and A. A. E. F. Saleh, "Early Prediction of Chronic Kidney Disease Using Deep Belief Network," in *IEEE Access*, vol. 9, pp. 135542–135549, 2021, DOI: 10.1109/ACCESS.2021.3114306.
32. X. Jiang, J. Zhao, W. Qian, W. Song and G. N. Lin, "A Generative Adversarial Network Model for Disease Gene Prediction With RNA-seq Data," in *IEEE Access*, vol. 8, pp. 37352–37360, 2020, DOI: 10.1109/ACCESS.2020.2975585.

# 4 Hybrid GAN Model with LSTM-Combined ResNet Discriminator for COVID-19 Classification in CT Images

*Somasundaram Krishnamoorthy, Sivakumar Paulraj, Sridevi Sriram, Baskaran Periyasamy, Sivaraman Eswaran, and Ramamoorthy Arun Kumar*

## 4.1 INTRODUCTION

The healthcare industry has been facing challenges in integrating vast amounts of diverse data from various sources Semantic Data Fabric (SDF) is a promising solution to this problem that uses artificial intelligence (AI) algorithms to automatically integrate and interpret complex healthcare data This technology can facilitate risk prognosis and preventive care. This chapter focuses on developing a Semantic Data Fabric for Automated Health Care Data Integration using AI for Risk Prognosis and Preventive Care, specifically targeting the challenges of prognosis tracking and adverse effect monitoring in cancer diseases.

The appearance of the novel COVID-19 disease caused by severe acute respiratory syndrome coronavirus 2 (SARS-CoV-2) caused a global health emergency [1]. Since its first detection in late 2019, COVID-19 has rapidly spread across countries, leading to significant morbidity and mortality worldwide. This virus is initially transferred through respiratory droplets and close contact, making it highly contagious and challenging to contain.

COVID-19 shows a wide spectrum of symptoms, ranging from mild respiratory illness to severe pneumonia and multi-organ failure [2]. The major signs include fever, coughing, and difficulty breathing, while some individuals may remain asymptomatic carriers, unknowingly transmitting the virus to others. The disease poses a significant burden to healthcare systems, with severe cases requiring intensive care support and specialized treatment.

 DOI: 10.1201/9781003449058-4

The impact of COVID-19 extends beyond public health, affecting various aspects of society, including the economy, education, and daily life [3]. Different controlling activities like lockdowns, social distancing, and frequent testing have been implemented by Governments to avoid the spread of COVID-19. Vaccine development and mass vaccination campaigns have also played a crucial role in controlling the pandemic and reducing its severity.

The diagnosis of COVID-19 primarily relies on laboratory testing, including molecular tests such as the reverse transcription-polymerase chain reaction (RT-PCR) to detect viral genetic material and serological tests to detect antibodies. Compared to other techniques, the image processing-based diagnosis gives promising results and supports timely prediction.

CT imaging-based diagnosis reaches a maximum level of accuracy in COVID-19 detection using CT scans [4]. CT imaging has been considered as a powerful tool in the analysis and valuation of COVID-19. It offers detailed cross-sectional images of the lungs, permitting the visualization of characteristic abnormalities associated with the disease. The abnormal pattern of lungs can be easily identified through the CT scans. CT imaging supports an automated system to categorize the lung images into normal and abnormal stages. By analyzing the CT images, these algorithms can extract relevant features, quantify the extent of lung involvement, and provide a quantitative assessment of disease severity [5].

There are many image processing techniques that have been developed for this detection. These techniques include different steps like image enhancement, segmentation, feature extraction, and classification. Image enhancement algorithms are used to improve the quality of CT images by reducing noise, enhancing contrast, and highlighting relevant structures. Segmentation algorithms separate the lung regions from the surrounding tissues, facilitating the isolation and analysis of abnormalities. Feature extraction algorithms capture specific characteristics of COVID-19-related lung lesions, such as texture patterns or spatial distribution. Finally, classification algorithms use extracted features to differentiate between normal and abnormal cases.

The development of image processing-based COVID-19 detection algorithms is playing a major role in disease detection. This algorithm integrates machine learning (ML) and deep learning (DL) to accurately classify the images. These algorithms optimize the speed and accuracy of COVID-19 analysis, especially in regions where access to molecular testing is limited or time-consuming.

In this chapter, a novel image processing-based COVID-19 detection algorithm based on a GAN model is proposed using CT scans. There are different models proposed in literature, but the proposed model integrates LSTM and ResNet architectures for accurate classification. This integration allows extraction of more relevant features from CT images and supports improved feature classification.

The remaining portions of this chapter are arranged as follows: section 4.2 is the preliminaries of GAN and LSTM architectures. Section 4.3 summarizes related works. Section 4.4 presents the Hybrid GAN Model with LSTM-Combined ResNet Discriminator in detail and section 4.5 provides the results and discussion. Finally, Section 4.6 concludes the chapter.

## 4.2 PRELIMINARIES

### 4.2.1 GAN

Recently, GAN models have emerged as a powerful tool for image processing tasks. GANs consist of two important elements: a generator (G) and a discriminator (D), which work in parallel in a combative way to produce and evaluate synthetic images that closely resemble real images, as shown in Figure 4.1. This generation approach is used for different image processing tasks such as segmentation, restoration, and classification, especially in medical field.

The basic strategy behind GANs is the ability to learn and to capture the underlying distribution of training images, enabling the generator network to generate new, realistic images that exhibit similar characteristics. The discriminator network acts as a critic, distinguishing between original and generated images. By the learning process, the G module strives to produce images that can fool the D module, while the discriminator aims to accurately differentiate between real and generated images. The major application of the GAN model is image-to-image translation and super-resolution conversion.

In the medical field, the GAN model is used for three major tasks. First, the GAN model is used for data augmentations. The data insufficiency problems in critical disease data sets are effectively solved by GAN models. It generates more images based on augmentation to balance the data set in images. Then, it supports accurate segmentation and classification.

The generator and discriminator portions of the GAN model are modified to perform classification and segmentation tasks. The insertion of fully connected layers and softmax layers in the GAN model allows for the classification task. These layers are pretrained for larger images to undertake classification.

### 4.2.2 ResNet

The Residual Network, also called ResNet, is a widely adopted DL model that has revolutionized image classification and recognition tasks. It was first developed by

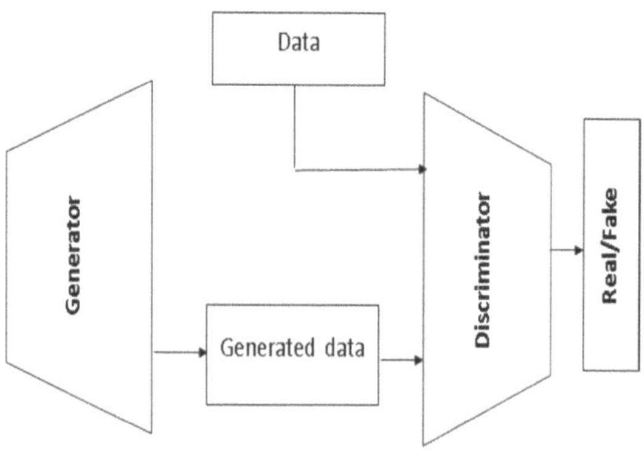


**FIGURE 4.1** GAN model.

Kaiming He et al. in 2015 and has since become a cornerstone in computer vision research.

The key major advantage of this type of network lies in its use of residual connections (RC) or skip connections (SC). These connections allow the network to learn residual mappings, making it easier to optimize and train DL models with hundreds or even thousands of layers. This is different to existing models, where increasing the network depth may lead to diminishing performance due to vanishing gradients.

The RC in ResNet allows information to flow directly across layers, preserving and propagating crucial information while avoiding degradation caused by DL models. To avoid the unnecessary processing of layers, the RC approach allows skip processing to learn the features. The model can focus on fine-tuning the residuals instead of directly learning the entire mapping by learning residuals.

ResNet introduces the concept of residual blocks RB, which consist of multiple layers. Each RB contains a set of convolutional layers followed by batch normalization and activation functions. The input to a RB is passed through the convolutional layers, and the output is added back to the original input using a skip connection. This skip connection ensures that the model can learn both the original features and the residual information simultaneously.

By cascading multiple RBs together, ResNet can effectively learn complex hierarchical features and capture intricate patterns within the data. The architecture of ResNet typically includes multiple stages, with each stage containing several RBs. The number of RBs and the depth of the network can be adjusted based on resource availability.

### 4.2.3 LSTM

LSTM is a modified version of a recurrent network which holds data in a memory unit for learning spatial features. The architecture of an LSTM model is shown in Figure 4.2. The major components of LSTM models are LSTM cells and gates.

The LSTM model takes input in the form of sequential data, such as time series data or text. The memory cells of the model help capture and retain information over long sequences. Each memory cell consists of three main components: an input gate (IG), a forget gate (FG), and an output gate (OG). The input gate is responsible for controlling the amount of data to be added to the memory cell. It decides data's importance by calculating the sigmoid functions between present and past input data. The forget gate is responsible for deleting unnecessary data to the next state. It decides on deletion by calculating the sigmoid of present and past hidden state values. The functions of gate outputs and LSTM outputs can be seen below in Equations (9.1) to (9.8):

$$f_t = \sigma\left(W_{xf}.x_t + .W_{hf}.h_t - 1 + b_f\right) \tag{9.1}$$

$$i_t = \sigma\left(W_{xi}.x_t + .W_{hi}.h_t - 1 + b_i\right) \tag{9.2}$$

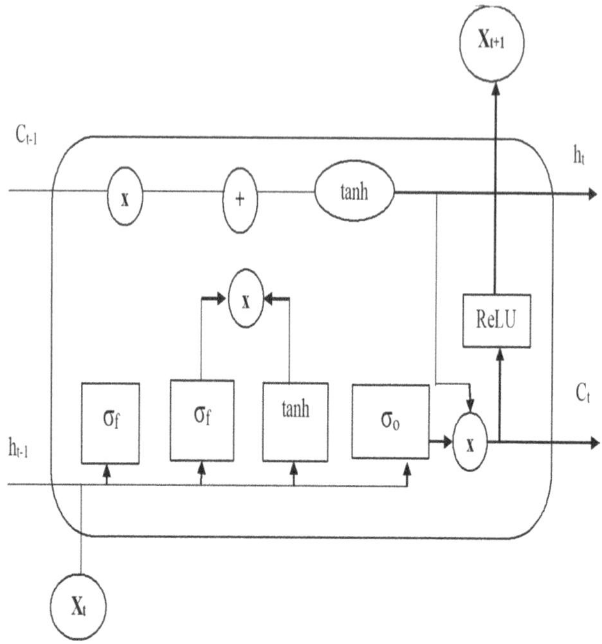


**FIGURE 4.2** LSTM architecture.

$$\overline{c}_t = tanh\left(W_{xc}.x_t + .W_{hc}.h_t - 1 + b_c\right) \tag{9.3}$$

$$c_t = f_t * c_{t-1} + i_t * \overline{c}_t \tag{9.4}$$

$$O_t = \sigma\left(W_{xo}.x_t + W_{ho}.h_t - 1 + b_o\right) \tag{9.5}$$

$$h_t = O_t * tanh \tag{9.6}$$

$$y_t = \sigma\left(W_{hy}.h_t + b_y\right) \tag{9.7}$$

$$\sigma(x) = \frac{1}{1+e^{-x}} \tag{9.8}$$

where $f_t$, $i_t$, $O_t$ represents the FG, IG, and OG functions with weights of $W_{xf}$, $W_{xi}$, and $W_{xo}$, respectively. b represents the bias values of activation functions

The cell state represents the long-term memory of the module. It is updated based on the IG and FG values. The current input, previous hidden state, and the gates' outputs are combined to update the cell state using a tanh activation function. The output gate controls the information to be passed from the memory cell to the output. It decides on deletion by calculating sigmoid of present and past hidden state values. The hidden state is the output of the LSTM cell and represents the short-term memory or the relevant information extracted from the input sequence. It is computed based on the updated cell state and the output gate. The LSTM model is trained using a labeled dataset through backpropagation. The parameters of the LSTM, including the weights and biases, are adjusted iteratively to minimize a defined loss function. This process allows the LSTM to learn patterns and relationships within the sequential data. By utilizing memory cells and capturing long-term dependencies, LSTM models are particularly effective in tasks involving sequential or time-dependent data.

## 4.3 RELATED WORK

Numerous research groups have conducted significant studies in the field of medical image processing, focusing on various aspects of this domain. In this section, a summary of selected works conducted by researchers in the segmentation and classification algorithms are provided, highlighting their key findings and contributions.

K. Sun et al. [6] developed a convolutional neural network architecture for COVID-19 detection with high accuracy. The developed architecture uses a residual network to reduce the computation cost of the training model without compromising the accuracy level. The accuracy achieved by the proposed model is about 98.5%, which is better than the previously developed models. A hybrid CNN model combined with data augmentation technique is proposed by W. Sae-Lim et al. [7] for categorizing the COVID-19 CT images based on the severity level. The data augmentation technique is applied to increase the feature extraction capability of the model without increasing network complexity. Also, the Gradient-weighted Class Activation Mapping approach is used to improve the processing of CT images.

Y. Pathak et al. [8] proposed a bidirectional deep learning model for classification. The proposed model combines a mixture density network to process the feature on both sides. The parameter of the model is tuned using memetic differential optimization algorithms. Compared to the model without optimization, the mixture network model shows higher accuracy with proper parameter tuning.

Acombined segmentation and classification model was introduced by Y. -H. Wu et al. [9]. The concept of attention mechanism is applied to increase the feature learning capacity of the model. The proposed model was verified on public CT image data sets and achieved an accuracy result of 94.5%, which is higher than existing learning models.

To improve the classification accuracy, a hybrid model was proposed by N. L. I. Huda et al. [10] which combines advantages of both machine learning and deep models. The proposed classification system performs two key operations: histogram-oriented feature extraction and classification using a Support Vector Machine (SVM) integrated with a DarkNet model. Results on CT image data set show that the hybrid model reaches a maximum accuracy of 97.8 for all cases. The concept of vector quantization was used by L. Trinh et al. [11] for COVID-19 classification. It uses a finite set of vectors for the classification of images. The vector quantization also supports training the model with a minimum number of images. The model shows a higher accuracy with a minimum training rate.

J. Li, D. Zhang, et al. [12] constructed a new hybrid learning model for COVID-19 CT image processing. This model combines a ResNet model with a graph attention network for classification. The graph attention network assigns attention coefficients to different pairs of pixels to process the images. The complexity of the models is slightly increased with the integration of the attention network.

The concept of transfer learning (TL) is introduced to share the knowledge between two models to increase a learning capacity of the models. This TL approach was used by M. I. Daoud et al. [13] to classify the COVID-19 images. The U-Net is combined with GoogleNet for transfer learning and to categorize the images into normal and abnormal stages. An average accuracy of 95.9% is reached by the utilization of TL in classification.

Y. Shi et al. [14] proposed a DL model-based channel attention mechanism for classification. This channel attention is used to assign a weight for features in feature mapping. Also, the important features were considered for feature selection process. For classification, the DenseNet model is used.

Acombined model of SVM and CNN for lung CT image classification was introduced by S. Al-Jumaili et al. [15]. The nonlinearity in pixel intensity is effectively handled by SVM and features are effectively represented using CNN. This combination increases overall accuracy of the model. M. E. Irawati et al. [16] proposed a fusion model for COVID-19 classification. The features are extracted using a k means algorithm. The features from the k means algorithm and hue features are fused to get a final important feature. The AdaBoost classifier is used for final classification. Compared to the existing model, the fusion-based model shows a higher accuracy of 96.89%.

The texture features play a major role in the field of medical image classification. The different texture features are Gray-Level Co-occurrence Matrix (GLCM), Local Binary Patterns (LBP), Histogram of Oriented Gradients (HOG), Local Binary Patterns on Three Orthogonal Planes (LBP-TOP), Tamura Features, and Haralick Features. These features reflect the spatial features of the image for accurate detection. A texture feature-based lung CT image classification was proposed by L. N. Rohmah et al. [17] for COVID-19. The features are classified using an SVM algorithm. The evaluation results show that the consideration of texture features can provide accuracy up to 96.4% on CT images.

Y. Jusman et al. [18] proposed a COVID-19 classification algorithm by combining three different ML models. The features are extracted using wavelet transform. Then, the disease severity is classified by combining SVM, AdaBoost, and random forest algorithms. The proposed models show a best result with an accuracy of 79.8%.

To improve the performance of classification, the results of different learning models are combined in ensemble models. The strategy of ensemble models is used for lung image processing by T. B. Saputra et al. [19] to classify the pneumonia disease. The DL models of VGG, GoogleNet, and mobile net are used for classification and soft voting is applied for decision-making.

The modified CNN model was developed by D. Reynaldi et al. [20] for classifying normal and abnormal cases in a COVID-19 image data set. Initially, the images are pre-processed using adaptive histogram equalization. Then, the layer modified CNN is applied for feature learning and classification. The adaptive histogram equalization supports improved model accuracy by handling noise effectively. To overcome the problem of data set insufficiency, the GAN-based image generation model was applied by Z. Liang et al. [21] for chest X-ray image classification. An additional 1256 images are generated using a GAN model to tackle the insufficiency of the data set. For classification, the layer modified ResNet is used. The accuracy level is increased by about 3.55% when using a GAN model for classification.

A new encoder-decoder-encoder architecture was proposed by X. Zhang et al.[22] for lung disease classification in CT images. The additional encoder in the DL model improves the feature extraction property of the model and supports computation minimization. The overall processing cost of the learning model is reduced when compared to other learning models. A modified CNN model named CovidNet was developed by A. Al–Monsur et al. [23].An ensemble learning layer is added to a VGG model to construct CovidNet. The VGG model without an ensemble layer reaches an accuracy of 94.5%, but the model with an ensemble layer reaches an accuracy of 96.58%.

Combined TL and optimization were used by Y. Wang et al. [24] to classify the lung disease for the CT image data base. The TL is used in VGG architecture for classification. Also, the Squeeze attention mechanism is used to increase the performance of the TL model. The parameters of the TL model are tuned at run time to increase accuracy.

A two-step classification model was proposed by S. Al-Jumaili et al. [25] for-X-ray image processing. As a first step, the features like LBP are extracted in X-ray images. Then, the SVM classifier is used for classification. M. Yamaç et al. [26] presented a convolution support estimation network to classify pneumonia in X-ray images. For pre-processing, a median filter is used. The classification is done by an AdaBoost classifier.

## 4.4 PROPOSED MODEL

The proposed GAN model in this chapter introduces a novel combination of an LSTM-based generator and a ResNet-based discriminator, aiming to enhance the quality and fidelity of generated images while improving the discrimination between real and generated images, as shown in Figure 4.3.

The LSTM-based generator is designed to effectively model sequential dependencies within the input data. This is particularly valuable for tasks where the temporal coherence of the generated images is crucial. Due to the recurrent nature of LSTM, the generator can capture long-term dependencies and generate coherent sequences of image features. This enables the model to produce more realistic and visually consistent images compared to traditional generator architectures.

Complementing the LSTM-based generator, the ResNet-based discriminator offers effective discriminative capabilities to the GAN model. By using ResNet in the discriminator, the model can effectively differentiate between real and generated CT lung images, discriminating even refined differences in image quality and authenticity.

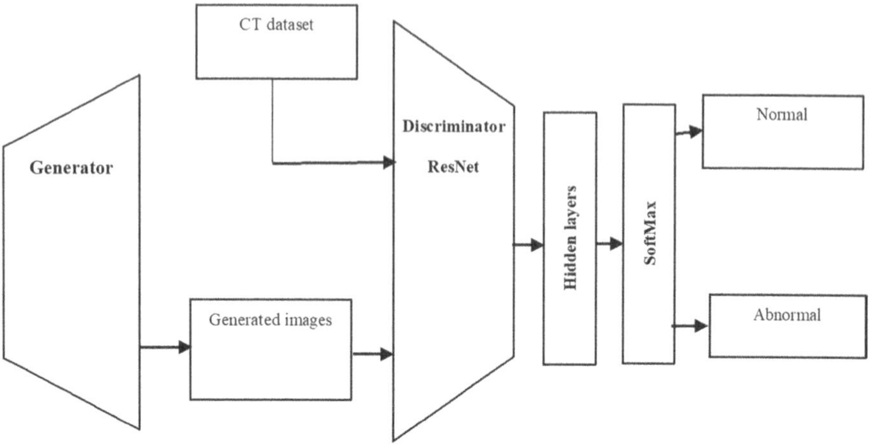


**FIGURE 4.3** Proposed GAN model.

Through the iterative training process, the module G continuously improves its ability to generate CT images, while the module D becomes increasingly proficient in differentiating between real and generated samples.

By combining the strengths of LSTM and ResNet within the GAN architecture, the proposed model offers a unique advantage in disease classification. It can generate representation that not only exhibits temporal coherence and realistic features but also passes the scrutiny of a highly discriminative discriminator. This leads to the effective classification of lung disease. In the proposed GAN model with ResNet as the discriminator, the loss functions can be represented using equations.

Adversarial Loss (Generator Loss): The module G loss encourages the G network to generate samples that are classified as real by the D module. It is computed using the binary cross-entropy loss, comparing the discriminator's output for generated samples (D(G(z))) with the target label of "real" (1) as in Equation (9.9).

$$\text{Generator Loss} = -\log(D(G(z))) \tag{9.9}$$

Adversarial Loss + Regularizer (Discriminator Loss):

The discriminator loss aims to maximize the differentiating ability to correctly classify real and generated samples. It consists of two portions: the adversarial loss and a regularizer term. The adversarial loss compares the D modules output for real samples (D(x)) with the target label of "real" (1) and the D modules output for created samples (D(G(z))) with the target label of "fake" (0). The regularizer term can include additional components to stabilize the training process as in Equation (9.10).

$$\text{Discriminator Loss} = -\log(D(x)) - \log(1 - D(G(z))) + \text{Regularizer Term} \tag{9.10}$$

The regularizer term can vary depending on the specific requirements of the GAN model. It may include additional loss components such as gradient penalties, label smoothing, or regularization terms to increase the stability and performance of the training. The pseudo code for the proposed model is given below:

```
# Generator (LSTM)
def generator(input):
    # Define LSTM layers
    lstm_layer_1 = LSTM(units=hidden_units_1, return_sequences=True)(input)
    lstm_layer_2 = LSTM(units=hidden_units_2, return_sequences=True)
(lstm_layer_1)
    # Additional LSTM layers
    # ...
    # Output layer
    generated_image=Dense(units=num_output_channels,activation='tanh')
(lstm_layer_2)
    return generated_image
  # Discriminator (ResNet)
  def discriminator(input):
    # Define ResNet layers
    resnet_layer_1 = ResNetBlock(input)
    resnet_layer_2 = ResNetBlock(resnet_layer_1)
    # Additional ResNet layers
    # ...
    # Output layer
    classification = Dense(units=1, activation='sigmoid')(resnet_layer_2)
    return classification
  # Combined GAN model
  def gan_model(generator, discriminator):
    # Freeze the discriminator weights during GAN training
    discriminator.trainable = False
    # GAN input
    gan_input = Input(shape=input_shape)
    # Generate image using generator
    generated_image = generator(gan_input)
    # Get classification prediction using discriminator
    gan_output = discriminator(generated_image)
    # GAN model
    gan = Model(inputs=gan_input, outputs=[generated_image, gan_output])
    return gan
  # Define loss functions and optimizers
  gan_model.compile(loss=['mse', 'binary_crossentropy'], optimizer=gan_
optimizer)
  # Training loop
  epoch = 0
  while epoch < num_epochs:
    # Generate fake images
    generated_images = generator.predict(real_images)
    # Combine real and fake images for discriminator training
```

```
        combined_images = np.concatenate([real_images, generated_images])
        # Labels for images
        labels = np.concatenate([np.ones((batch_size, 1)), np.zeros((batch_
    size, 1))])
        # Train discriminator
        discriminator_loss = discriminator_model.train_on_batch(combined_
    images, labels)
        # Train generator
        gan_loss = gan_model.train_on_batch(real_images, [real_images,
    np.ones((batch_size, 1))])
        # Print loss and accuracy metrics for monitoring
        # Increment epoch counter
        epoch += 1
      # Evaluate the trained GAN model on test data
      Parameter tuning using optimizer
```

The Aquila Optimizer (AO) is a population-based optimization algorithm inspired by the behavior of the Aquila bird during the process of catching prey. The algorithm aims to efficiently explore and exploit the solution space to find optimal solutions for various optimization problems. The AO algorithm is organized into four stages:

### 4.4.1 Selecting the Search Space by High Soar with Vertical Stoop

In this phase, the algorithm performs a high soar to select the search space and then employs a vertical stoop to rapidly descend into a promising area. The high soar allows the algorithm to explore the solution space from a broader perspective, while the vertical stoop allows it to rapidly dive into regions with potential optimal solutions as in Equation (9.11).

$$X_1'(t'+1) = X_{best}'(t') \times \left(1 - \frac{1}{T}\right) + \left(X_M'(t') - X_{best}'(t')^* r\right) \tag{9.11}$$

where Xi, X´M, and $X'_{best}$ are the different locations of aquila based on movements.

### 4.4.2 Exploring Within a Diverge Search Space by Contour Flight with Short Glide Attack

During this phase, the algorithm engages in contour flight to explore within a diverging search space. The contour flight enables it to navigate through various regions of the search space, while the short glide attack allows it to perform focused exploration in the vicinity of potential solutions. The updated position is computed as in Equation (9.12):

$$X_2'(t'+1) = X_{best}'(t') \times \text{levy}(D) + X_R'(t') + (y' - x')^* r \tag{9.12}$$

### 4.4.3 Exploiting Within a Converge Search Space by Low Flight with Slow Descent Attack

In this phase, the algorithm performs a low flight to exploit within a converging search space. The low flight helps the algorithm focus on local regions with higher potential for optimal solutions, while the slow descent attack allows it to fine-tune and improve the solutions in those regions. The updated position is computed as in Equation (9.13):

$$X_3'\left(t'+1\right)=X_{best}'\left(t'\right)-X_M'\left(t'\right)\times\propto'-r+\left(\left(UB'-LB'\right)\times r+LB'\right)\times\delta' \quad (9.13)$$

### 4.4.4 Swooping by Walk and Grab Prey

During the final phase, the algorithm swoops by employing a walk and grab prey approach. It leverages the information gathered during the previous phases to converge towards the most promising solutions in the search space. The updated position is computed as in Equation (9.14):

$$X_4'\left(t'+1\right)=QF'\times X_{best}'\left(t'\right)\times\left(G_1'\times X'\left(t\right)\times r\right)-G_2'\times levy\left(D\right)+r\times G_1' \quad (9.14)$$

### 4.4.5 Hyperparameter Tuning AO

The hyperparameters of the GAN model include Kernel Size, Stride, Padding, Number of Filters and Activation Function and Pooling, Pooling layers and average-pooling layers. These hyperparameters are tuned to find the optimal combination that yields the best performance of the GAN model on COVID-19 prediction. Hyperparameter tuning is essential to avoid overfitting or underfitting the model, achieve better generalization, and improve overall model performance. In this chapter, the hyperparameters are tuned using AO. The pseudocode for parameter tuning using AO is given below:

```
# Aquila Optimizer pseudocode for tuning GAN hyperparameters
def aquila_optimizer_gan(num_aquilas, max_generations, ul, ll):
  # Initialize the swarm of aquilas with random positions
  swarm = initialize_swarm(num_aquilas, ul, ll)
    for generation in range(max_generations):
    for aquila in swarm:
      # Phase 1: Random Movement
      P_new = random_movement(aquila.position, ul, ll)
      fitness = evaluate_gan_fitness(P_new)
      if fitness < aquila.best_fitness:
          aquila.best_position = P_new
          aquila.best_fitness = fitness
          # Phase 2: Fighting
    for i in range(1, num_aquilas):
      P_new = chain_movement(swarm[i].position, swarm[i - 1].position)
```

```
            fitness = evaluatc_gan_fitness(P_new)
            if fitness < swarm[i].best_fitness:
                swarm[i].best_position = P_new
                swarm[i].best_fitness = fitness
                # Phase 3: Adjusting Position
        leaders = select_group_leaders(swarm)
        for aquila in swarm:
            P_new = leader_adjustment(aquila.position, best_leader_position(leaders))
            fitness = evaluate_gan_fitness(P_new)
            if fitness < aquila.best_fitness:
                aquila.best_position = P_new
                aquila.best_fitness = fitness
    # Phase 4: Leading the Group by the Leaders Towards the Optimal Area (Leader Movement)
            update_leader_positions(leaders)
            # Return the best hyperparameter set found in the swarm
        best_aquila = min(swarm, key=lambda x: x.best_fitness)
        return best_aquila.best_position
```

## 4.5 RESULTS AND DISCUSSION

The dataset used in this study was obtained from the Kaggle website (https://github.com/mr7495/COVID-CTset). It consists of a comprehensive collection of original CT scans from 377 individuals. The dataset comprises a total of 59,756 CT scan images, with 16,470 images belonging to 89 patients diagnosed with COVID-19 and 37,654 images from 393 individuals classified as normal cases. The CT scans were acquired at the Negin medical center located in Sari, Iran, using a SOMATOM Scope model. The radiology images were exported in an 8-bit grayscale DICOM format with a resolution of 512x512 pixels. The sample data set image is shown in Figure 4.4.

The pre-processed and segmented images are shown in Figure 4.5. The performance of the proposed model was analyzed in terms of Precision, Recall, Accuracy, F1 score, Root Mean Squared Error (RMSE), and Mean Absolute Error (MAE). The above parameters can be obtained by substituting true positives (TP), false positives (FP), false negatives (FN), and true negatives (TN) of the results, as in Equations (9.15) to (9.20).

$$\text{Precision } (\%) = (TP / (TP + FP)) * 100 \tag{9.15}$$

$$\text{Recall } (\%) = (TP / (TP + FN)) * 100 \tag{9.16}$$

$$\text{Accuracy } (\%) = ((TP + TN) / (TP + TN + FP + FN)) * 100 \tag{9.17}$$

$$\text{F1 score } (\%) = (2 * \text{Precision} * \text{Recall}) / (\text{Precision} + \text{Recall}) * 100 \tag{9.18}$$

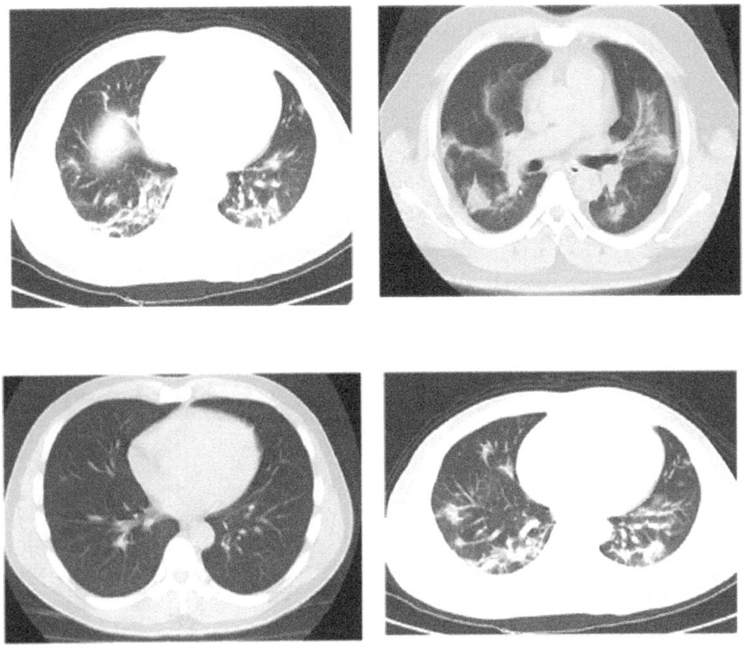

**FIGURE 4.4** Data set images.

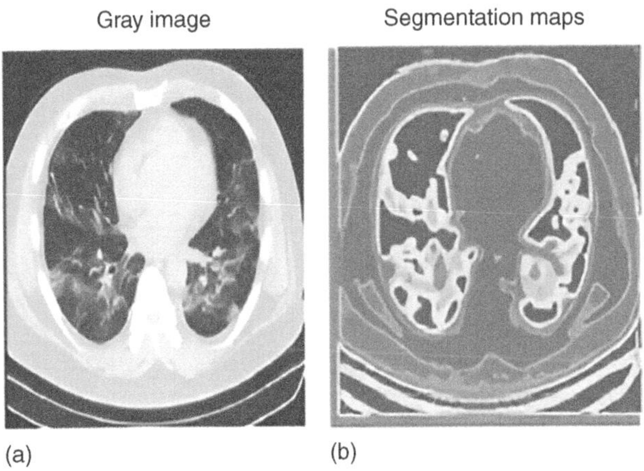


**FIGURE 4.5** Processed images.

$$\text{RMSE} = \text{sqrt}((1/N) * \text{sum}((\text{predicted - actual})\text{^}2)) \tag{9.19}$$

$$\text{MAE} = (1/N) * \text{sum}(\text{abs}(\text{predicted - actual})) \tag{9.20}$$

The layer training and evaluated accuracy results of proposed model are visualized in Figure 4.6.

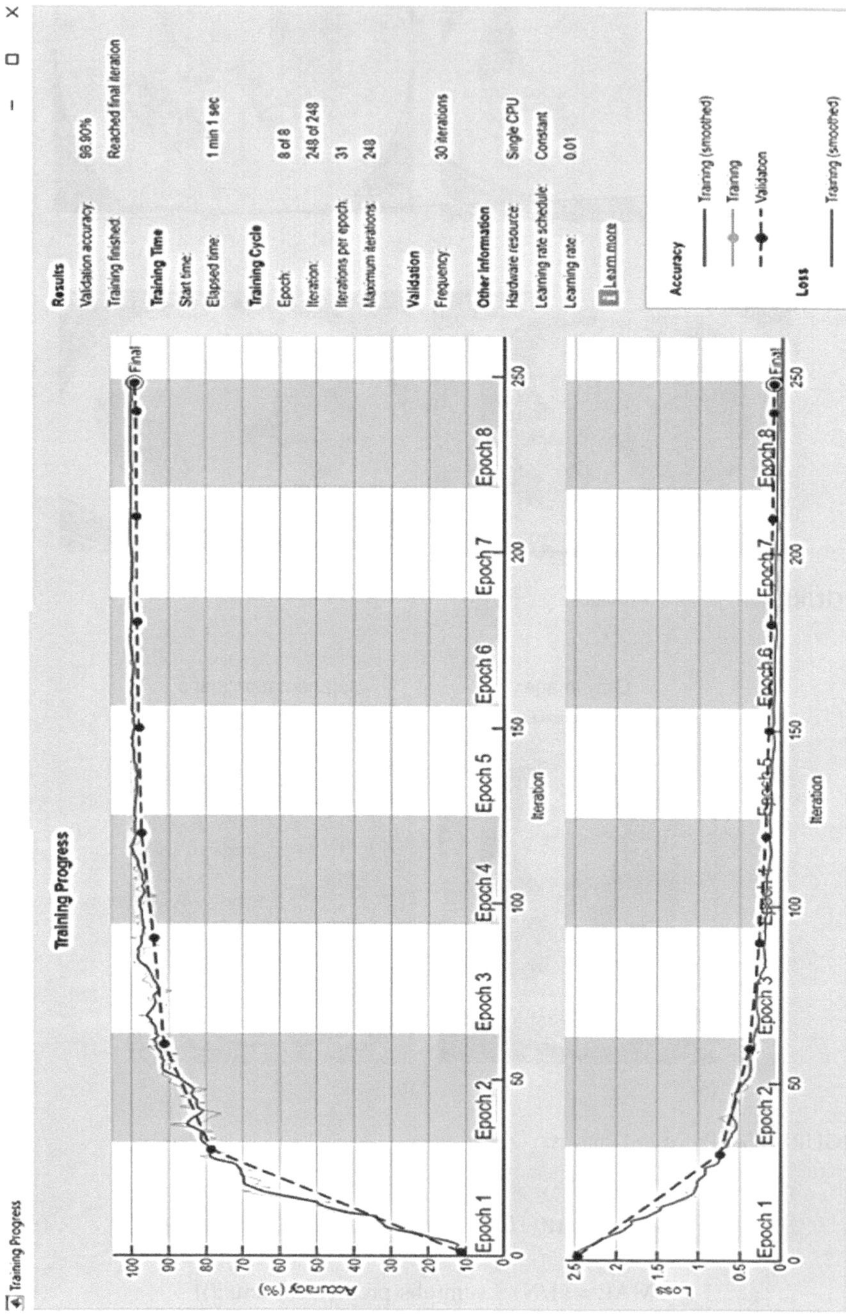


FIGURE 4.6 Model evaluation and training.

**TABLE 4.1**
**Performance Evaluation**

| Techniques | Precision (%) | Recall (%) | Accuracy (%) | F1 score (%) |
|---|---|---|---|---|
| Hybrid GAN with LSTM | 99.2 | 98.9 | 98.9 | 99.1 |
| Stack GAN | 97.5 | 96.85 | 96.59 | 96.7 |
| ResNet | 96.12 | 95.2 | 95.9 | 94.25 |
| GoogleNet | 95.2 | 95.6 | 95 | 93.42 |
| Modified U-Net | 93 | 94.12 | 94.32 | 92.8 |
| BPNN | 92.85 | 93.55 | 93.2 | 91.8 |
| CNN | 91.695 | 92.44 | 92.85 | 89.23 |
| ANN | 90.5 | 91.24 | 91.9 | 88.65 |

The measure results of proposed model are given in Table 4.1. The Hybrid GAN with LSTM model demonstrates exceptional performance, achieving a precision of 99.2%, indicating its ability to accurately classify positive cases. Moreover, it attains a recall rate of 98.9%, suggesting its effectiveness in correctly identifying a large proportion of actual positives. The model's high accuracy of 98.9% reflects its overall correctness in predicting both positive and negative cases. Additionally, the F1 score of 99.1% highlights the model's ability to strike a balance between precision and recall, proving its reliability in classification tasks.

Comparatively, other models such as Stack GAN, ResNet, GoogleNet, Modified U-Net, BPNN, CNN, and ANN also exhibit competitive performance across the evaluation metrics. Compared to other model results, the Hybrid GAN with LSTM model consistently outperforms them in all parameters. This shows the superior predictive capability and effectiveness of the Hybrid GAN with LSTM model in classification.

For instance, the Hybrid GAN with LSTM model showcases an increment of 1.68% in precision compared to the second-best model, Stack GAN. In terms of recall, it exhibits an increment of 2.05% over the nearest competitor, ResNet. Similarly, the model demonstrates an increment of 1.75% in accuracy compared to GoogleNet and achieves a remarkable increment of 3.91% in F1 score over ANN as shown in Figure 4.7.

The Hybrid GAN with LSTM technique demonstrates a remarkable precision of 99.2%, proving its superior performance in COVID-19 detection. When compared to other models, the incremental percentage of precision highlights its significant advantages. Compared to the Stack GAN model, the Hybrid GAN with LSTM achieves an impressive 1.7% increase in precision, indicating its enhanced ability to accurately identify COVID-19. Moreover, when compared to other models like ResNet and GoogleNet, the Hybrid GAN with LSTM exhibits a notable incremental percentage of 3.08% and 4%, respectively, further supporting its effectiveness in achieving precise and reliable detection results. The incremental percentage signifies the tangible improvement provided by the Hybrid GAN with LSTM approach, making it a promising approach in the field of COVID-19 detection.

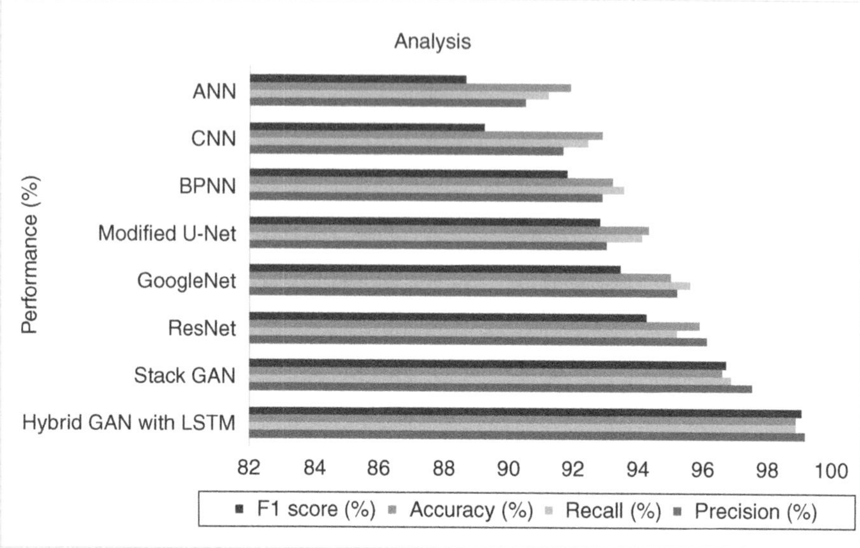


**FIGURE 4.7** The performance of the proposed GAN model.

The Hybrid GAN with LSTM technique proves an impressive recall rate of 98.9% in COVID-19 detection, highlighting its superior performance. When compared to other models, the incremental percentage of recall proves its advantages. Compared to the Stack GAN model, the Hybrid GAN with LSTM shows a substantial increase of 2.05% in recall, indicating its enhanced ability to identify true positive cases of COVID-19. Similarly, when compared to widely used models like ResNet and GoogleNet, the Hybrid GAN with LSTM exhibits incremental percentages of 3.7% and 3.3%, respectively, proving its superior recall performance. Additionally, compared to the Modified U-Net model, the Hybrid GAN with LSTM achieves a significant 4.78% incremental percentage, further establishing its efficacy in accurately detecting COVID-19. These incremental percentages signify the valuable improvement provided by the Hybrid GAN with LSTM approach, making it a reliable and promising technique in the field of COVID-19 detection.

The Hybrid GAN with LSTM technique stands out with an impressive accuracy of 98.9% in COVID-19 detection, proving its superior performance. A comparison with other models reveals substantial incremental percentages in accuracy. When compared to the Stack GAN model, the Hybrid GAN with LSTM shows a notable increase of 2.31%, underscoring its enhanced accuracy in identifying COVID-19. Moreover, compared to widely used models like ResNet and GoogleNet, the Hybrid GAN with LSTM exhibits incremental percentages of 3% and 3.9%, respectively, further emphasizing its superior accuracy. Additionally, when compared to the Modified U-Net model, the Hybrid GAN with LSTM demonstrates a significant incremental percentage of 4.58%, reinforcing its ability to provide precise and reliable detection results. These incremental percentages highlight the valuable improvement offered by

**TABLE 4.2**
**Performance Evaluation**

| Techniques | RMSE | MAE |
|---|---|---|
| Hybrid GAN with LSTM | 1.115 | 1.845 |
| Stack GAN | 3.426 | 3.142 |
| ResNet | 3.751 | 3.766 |
| GoogleNet | 4.211 | 4.842 |
| Modified U-Net | 4.043 | 4.860 |
| BPNN | 5.175 | 5.978 |
| CNN | 5.458 | 6.265 |
| ANN | 5.956 | 7.23 |

the Hybrid GAN with LSTM technique, establishing it as a promising and effective approach for accurate COVID-19 detection.

The Hybrid GAN with LSTM technique outperforms other models by achieving a high F1 score, signifying its superior performance in accurately detecting COVID-19. When compared to the Stack GAN model, it shows a noteworthy incremental percentage of 2.4%, demonstrating its enhanced ability to strike a balance between precision and recall. Additionally, compared to widely used models like ResNet and GoogleNet, the Hybrid GAN with LSTM exhibits incremental percentages of 4.85% and 5.68%, respectively, indicating its improved capability in providing accurate and reliable COVID-19 detection. Furthermore, compared to the Modified U-Net model, the Hybrid GAN with LSTM provides a substantial incremental percentage of 6.3%, reinforcing its effectiveness in achieving precise and robust detection results.

The performance results based on error rate are given in Table 4.2. When comparing the performance of the Hybrid GAN with LSTM model to other models based on the provided RMSE and MAE metrics, there are interesting results in prediction accuracy.

The Hybrid GAN with LSTM model stands out with significantly lower RMSE and MAE values, indicating its superior performance in minimizing the average squared differences and absolute differences between predicted and actual values, respectively. With an RMSE of 1.115 and MAE of 1.845, the model demonstrates its ability to provide highly accurate predictions with minimal errors.

In contrast, other models such as Stack GAN, ResNet, GoogleNet, Modified U-Net, BPNN, CNN, and ANN exhibit relatively higher RMSE and MAE values, suggesting higher prediction errors and less precision in estimating the target variable.

For instance, compared to the second-best model, Stack GAN, the Hybrid GAN with LSTM model showcases a decrement of 67.54% in RMSE and 41.46% in MAE. Similarly, it exhibits a decrement of 64.36% in RMSE and 36.58% in MAE compared to ANN, the model with the highest values in these metrics, as shown in Figure 4.8.

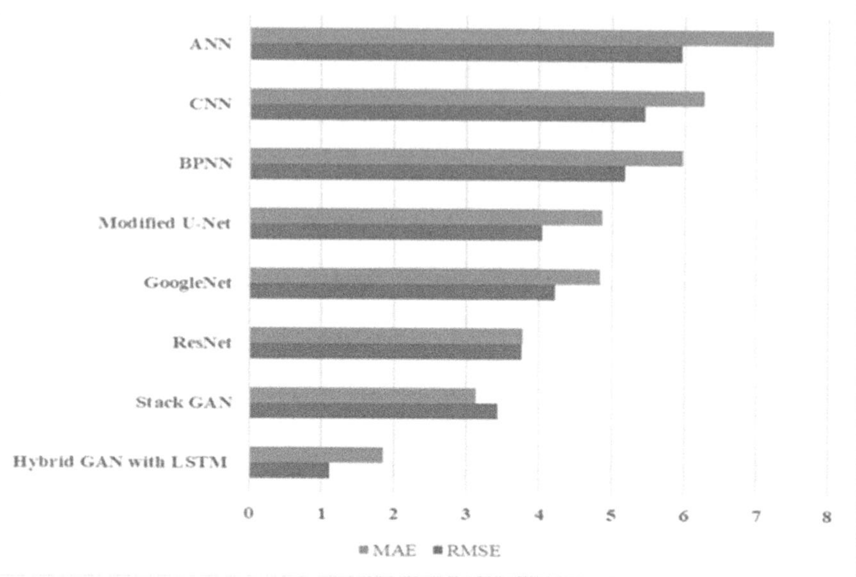


**FIGURE 4.8** Error rate analysis.

## 4.6 CONCLUSION

The Hybrid GAN with LSTM model demonstrates superior results with an RMSE of 1.115 and MAE of 1.845, indicating its capability to produce predictions with high accuracy and low errors. In contrast, the other models show larger errors, showcasing their limitations in precision. The Stack GAN, while offering competitive performance compared to other models, exhibits a noticeable decrease in precision with an RMSE of 3.426 and MAE of 3.142. This corresponds to a significant percentage decrease of approximately 67.463% in RMSE and 57.078% in MAE compared to the Hybrid GAN with LSTM model. The ResNet and GoogleNet models also show larger errors, with RMSE values of 3.751 and 4.211, and MAE values of 3.766 and 4.842, respectively. The Modified U-Net, BPNN, CNN, and ANN models further demonstrate higher errors, emphasizing the Hybrid GAN with LSTM model's superior performance.

## REFERENCES

1. WHO. Coronavirus Disease (COVID-19) Outbreak Situation, 2020. [Online]. Available: www.who.int/emergencies/diseases/novelcoronavirus-2019 www.who.int/emergencies/diseases/novel-coronavirus-2019
2. H. B. Jenssen. China National Health Commission Diagnosis and Treatment of Pneumonitis Caused by New Coronavirus (Trial Version 6). Accessed: Sep. 8, 2020. [Online]. Available: www.nhc.gov.cn/yzygj/s7653p/202002/8334a8326dd94d329df351d7da8ae % fc2.shtml

3. T. Ai et al., "Correlation of Chest CT and RT-PCR Testing in Coronavirus Disease 2019 (COVID-19) in China: A Report of 1014 Cases," in *Radiology*, vol. 296, no. 2, pp. E32–E40, 2020.
4. Y. Fang et al., "Sensitivity of Chest CT for COVID-19: Comparison to RT-PCR," in *Radiology*, vol. 296, no. 2, pp. E115–E117, Aug. 2020.
5. Y. Wang, H. Hou, W. Wang, and W. Wang, "Combination of CT and RT-PCR in the screening or diagnosis of COVID-19,"in *Journal of Global Health*, vol. 10, no. 1, pp. 1–4, Jun. 2020.
6. K. Sun, J. Zhu, H. Yuan, D. Li, C. Wang and Z. Wang, "CT Image Classification and Detection of COVID-19 Based on Convolutional Neural Network,"2021 IEEE International Conference on Recent Advances in Systems Science and Engineering (RASSE), Shanghai, China, 2021, pp. 1–5, doi: 10.1109/RASSE53195.2021.9686902.
7. W. Sae-Lim, R. Suwannanon and P. Aiyarak, "A Simplified Convolutional Neural Network Design for COVID-19 Classification on Chest X-ray Images,"2022 19th International Joint Conference on Computer Science and Software Engineering (JCSSE), Bangkok, Thailand, 2022, pp. 1–6, doi: 10.1109/JCSSE54890.2022.9836299.
8. Y. Pathak, P. K. Shukla and K. V. Arya, "Deep Bidirectional Classification Model for COVID-19 Disease Infected Patients," in *IEEE/ACM Transactions on Computational Biology and Bioinformatics*, vol. 18, no. 4, pp. 1234–1241, 1 July-Aug. 2021, doi: 10.1109/TCBB.2020.3009859.
9. Y. -H. Wu et al., "JCS: An Explainable COVID-19 Diagnosis System by Joint Classification and Segmentation," in *IEEE Transactions on Image Processing*, vol. 30, pp. 3113–3126, 2021,doi: 10.1109/TIP.2021.3058783.
10. N. L. I. Huda, M. A. Islam, M. O. Goni and N. Begum, "Covid-19 Classification Using HOG-SVM and Deep Learning Models,"2022 2nd International Conference on Innovative Research in Applied Science, Engineering and Technology (IRASET), Meknes, Morocco, 2022, pp. 1–5, doi: 10.1109/IRASET52964.2022.9738357.
11. L. Trinh, B. Ha and A. T. Tran, "VQC-COVID-NET: Vector Quantization Contrastive Learning for Covid-19 Image Base Classification,"2022 9th NAFOSTED Conference on Information and Computer Science (NICS), Ho Chi Minh City, Vietnam, 2022, pp. 247–251, doi: 10.1109/NICS56915.2022.10013439.
12. J. Li, D. Zhang, Q. Liu, R. Bu and Q. Wei, "COVID-GATNet: A Deep Learning Framework for Screening of COVID-19 from Chest X-Ray Images,"2020 IEEE 6th International Conference on Computer and Communications (ICCC), Chengdu, China, 2020, pp. 1897–1902, doi: 10.1109/ICCC51575.2020.9345005.
13. M. I. Daoud, Y. Alrahahleh, S. Abdel-Rahman, B. A. Alsaify and R. Alazrai, "COVID-19 Diagnosis in Chest X-ray Images by Combining Pre-trained CNN Models with Flat and Hierarchical Classification Approaches,"2021 12th International Conference on Information and Communication Systems (ICICS), Valencia, Spain, 2021, pp. 330–335, doi: 10.1109/ICICS52457.2021.9464532.
14. Y. Shi, T. Zhou, Z. You, J. Chu and T. Li, "AM-DenseNet: A Novel DenseNet Framework Using Attention Mechanisms for COVID-19 CT Image Classification,"2022 IEEE 8th International Conference on Cloud Computing and Intelligent Systems (CCIS), Chengdu, China, 2022, pp. 474–479, doi: 10.1109/CCIS57298.2022.10016401.
15. S. Al-Jumaili, A. D. Duru and O. N. Uçan, "Covid-19 Ultrasound Image Classification Using SVM Based on Kernels Deduced from Convolutional Neural Network,"2021 5th International Symposium on Multidisciplinary Studies and Innovative Technologies (ISMSIT), Ankara, Turkey, 2021, pp. 429–433, doi: 10.1109/ISMSIT52890.2021.9604551.

16. M. E. Irawati and H. Zakaria, "Classification Model for Covid-19 Detection Through Recording of Cough Using XGboost Classifier Algorithm,"2021 International Symposium on Electronics and Smart Devices (ISESD), Bandung, Indonesia, 2021, pp. 1–5, doi: 10.1109/ISESD53023.2021.9501695.
17. L. N. Rohmah and A. Bustamam, "Improved Classification of Coronavirus Disease (COVID-19) Based on Combination of Texture Features using CT Scan and X-ray Images,"2020 3rd International Conference on Information and Communications Technology (ICOIACT), Yogyakarta, Indonesia, 2020, pp. 105–109, doi: 10.1109/ICOIACT50329.2020.9332123.
18. Y. Jusman, D. W. Mubarok, S. Riyadi and S. N. A. M. Kanafiah, "COVID-19 X-Ray Images Classification Using Support Vector Machine and K-Nearest Neighbor,"2022 9th International Conference on Information Technology, Computer, and Electrical Engineering (ICITACEE), Semarang, Indonesia, 2022, pp. 217–221, doi: 10.1109/ICITACEE55701.2022.9924124.
19. T. B. Saputra, N. T. B. Pasaribu, A. Gany, J. Hasugian and E. M. Sartika, "Multiclass Classification of COVID-19, Pneumonia, or Nornal Lungs Based on Chest X -Ray Images with Ensemble Deep Learning,"2022 FORTEI-International Conference on Electrical Engineering (FORTEI-ICEE), Riau, Indonesia, 2022, pp. 76–80, doi: 10.1109/FORTEI-ICEE57243.2022.9972884.
20. D. Reynaldi, B. S. Negara, S. Sanjaya and E. Satria, "COVID-19 Classification for Chest X-Ray Images Using Deep Learning and Resnet-101,"2021 International Congress of Advanced Technology and Engineering (ICOTEN), Taiz, Yemen, 2021, pp. 1–4, doi: 10.1109/ICOTEN52080.2021.9493431.
21. Z. Liang, J. X. Huang, J. Li and S. Chan, "Enhancing Automated COVID-19 Chest X-ray Diagnosis by Image-to-Image GAN Translation,"2020 IEEE International Conference on Bioinformatics and Biomedicine (BIBM), Seoul, Korea (South), 2020, pp. 1068–1071, doi: 10.1109/BIBM49941.2020.9313466.
22. X. Zhang et al., "CXR-Net: A Multitask Deep Learning Network for Explainable and Accurate Diagnosis of COVID-19 Pneumonia from Chest X-Ray Images," in *IEEE Journal of Biomedical and Health Informatics*, vol. 27, no. 2, pp. 980–991, Feb. 2023, doi: 10.1109/JBHI.2022.3220813.
23. A. Al–Monsur, M. R. Kabir, A. M. Ar–Rafi, M. M. Nishat and F. Faisal, "Covid-EnsembleNet: An Ensemble Based Approach for Detecting Covid-19 by Utilising Chest X-ray Images,"2022 IEEE World AI IoT Congress (AIIoT), Seattle, WA, USA, 2022, pp. 351–356, doi: 10.1109/AIIoT54504.2022.9817237.
24. Y. Wang, "A New Classification Method for COVID-19 CT Images Based on Transfer Learning and Attention Mechanism,"2022 16th ICME International Conference on Complex Medical Engineering (CME), Zhongshan, China, 2022, pp. 236–240, doi: 10.1109/CME55444.2022.10063276.
25. S. Al-Jumaili, A. Al-Azzawi, A. D. Duru and A. A. Ibrahim, "Covid-19 X-ray Image Classification Using SVM Based on Local Binary Pattern,"2021 5th International Symposium on Multidisciplinary Studies and Innovative Technologies (ISMSIT), Ankara, Turkey, 2021, pp. 383–387, doi: 10.1109/ISMSIT52890.2021.9604731.
26. M. Yamaç, M. Ahishali, A. Degerli, S. Kiranyaz, M. E. H. Chowdhury and M. Gabbouj, "Convolutional Sparse Support Estimator-Based COVID-19 Recognition from X-Ray Images," in *IEEE Transactions on Neural Networks and Learning Systems*, vol. 32, no. 5, pp. 1810–1820, May 2021, doi: 10.1109/TNNLS.2021.3070467.

# 5 Dynamic Weighted Ensemble Framework

*Srinivas Arukonda and*
*Ramalingaswamy Cheruku*

## 5.1 INTRODUCTION

In medical diagnosis [1,2], accurate and timely detection of diseases is paramount to ensure effective treatment and patient outcomes. Machine learning [3], and specifically ensemble learning techniques, has shown promising results in improving diagnostic accuracy by combining multiple models. However, designing an effective ensemble system [4] that optimally combines diverse classifiers while maintaining interpretability remains challenging [5]. This chapter introduces a novel approach that leverages the Teaching-Learning-Based Optimization (TLBO) algorithm to dynamically optimize the fitness for disease diagnosis. TLBO is a nature-inspired optimization algorithm inspired by classroom teaching and learning processes [6]. By integrating TLBO with ensemble learning, we aim to enhance the performance and robustness of the ensemble system, making it more adaptive to varying diagnostic scenarios.

Ensemble learning [7] is a technique that combines multiple base classifiers (models) to make predictions. The idea behind ensemble learning is that by combining different classifiers, the strengths of individual models can compensate for each other's weaknesses, resulting in improved overall performance.

## 5.2 BACKGROUND

Disease diagnosis [8] involves identifying the presence of specific medical conditions based on various clinical and biomedical parameters. Early diagnosis is important because otherwise there may be a high mortality rate for chronic diseases such as diabetes, cancer, and heart disease [9]. Traditional single-model diagnostic systems often struggle to achieve high accuracy, especially in complex and diverse medical datasets. Ensemble learning has emerged as a powerful technique to tackle this issue by combining the predictions of multiple base models, leading to improved performance and generalization.

DOI: 10.1201/9781003449058-5

## 5.3 MOTIVATION

While ensemble learning has shown great potential in disease diagnosis, the effectiveness of ensemble models largely depends on the diversity and quality of the base classifiers. To address this, we propose a dynamic weighted ensemble approach that not only leverages the diversity of base models but also adaptively adjusts the weights of accuracy and diversity of classifiers on each bootstrapped bag based on their performance. The motivation behind this approach is to create a flexible and robust ensemble system that can adapt to different diagnostic scenarios.

## 5.4 OBJECTIVES

The main objectives of this chapter are as follows:

- Develop a dynamic ensemble learning approach that leverages TLBO to optimize the fitness of the bag and improves the worst bag fitness by balancing the accuracy and diversity weights.
- Evaluate the proposed approach with entropy-based diversity measure on benchmarked disease diagnosis datasets such as the Pima Indian dataset (PID), Statlog Heart Data (SHD), and Wilson Breast Cancer (WBC) from the UCI machine learning repository and compare its performance with traditional ensemble techniques.
- Evaluate the proposed model performance with statistical tests and compare it with baseline models

## 5.5 DISEASE DIAGNOSIS AND ENSEMBLE LEARNING

In this section, we delve into the field of disease diagnosis and how ensemble learning techniques have been employed to improve diagnostic accuracy [10]. We explore the overview of disease diagnosis, the integration of ensemble learning in this context, and the challenges and limitations associated with utilizing ensemble approaches for disease diagnosis.

### 5.5.1 Disease Diagnosis Overview

#### 5.5.1.1 Importance of Early Detection and Accurate Diagnosis

Disease diagnosis is a critical aspect of healthcare, involving the identification of specific medical conditions in patients based on various clinical, laboratory, and imaging data. Early detection and accurate diagnosis are essential for effective and timely treatment, which can significantly impact patient outcomes and quality of life. Timely diagnosis allows medical professionals to initiate appropriate interventions, improve patient management, and prevent the progression of diseases.

#### 5.5.1.2 Types of Diseases and Diagnostic Challenges

Diseases can vary widely in their nature, origin, and complexity. Some diseases are well-defined and have straightforward diagnostic criteria, while others may present with overlapping symptoms and manifestations, making diagnosis challenging. Additionally, certain diseases may have heterogeneous subtypes or stages, further complicating the diagnostic process. The diversity of diseases and their varying diagnostic challenges underscore the need for robust and accurate diagnostic methods.

### 5.5.2 Introduction to Ensemble Learning Techniques

Ensemble learning is a machine learning paradigm that involves combining multiple individual models (base learners) to form a more accurate and reliable predictive model. Ensemble methods harness the 'wisdom of the crowd' by aggregating the predictions of diverse models, leveraging their complementary strengths to compensate for individual weaknesses [11]. Ensemble techniques can significantly improve generalization and reduce overfitting, making them well-suited for complex and uncertain medical datasets.

### 5.5.3 Advantages of Ensemble Methods for Disease Diagnosis

Ensemble methods offer several advantages in the context of disease diagnosis:

1. **Improved accuracy**: Ensembles often outperform individual base classifiers, resulting in higher diagnostic accuracy.
2. **Robustness**: Ensemble models are less sensitive to noise and outliers in the data, enhancing their robustness.
3. **Increased generalization**: Ensembles can generalize better to unseen data, enhancing their ability to handle new cases.
4. **Handling uncertainty**: Ensemble methods can quantify prediction uncertainty, providing clinicians with more reliable diagnostic probabilities.

### 5.5.4 Popular Ensemble Approaches in Medical Diagnosis

Several ensemble learning techniques have been successfully applied in disease diagnosis, including:

1. **Bagging**: Bootstrap Aggregating [12] involves training multiple base models on different bootstrap samples of the data and combining their predictions by majority voting (classification) or averaging (regression).
2. **Boosting**: Boosting [13] algorithms sequentially build base models, giving more weight to misclassified instances, leading to a more accurate ensemble.
3. **Stacking**: Stacking [14], also known as Stacked Generalization, is an ensemble learning technique that combines multiple base classifiers (or models) to improve overall predictive performance. Unlike other ensemble methods like bagging and boosting, stacking involves training a 'meta-model' on the predictions made by the base classifiers rather than directly combining their individual predictions.

## 5.6 CHALLENGES AND LIMITATIONS

### 5.6.1 Challenges in Disease Diagnosis and Ensemble Learning

Despite the benefits of ensemble learning in disease diagnosis, there are specific challenges:

1. **Interpretability**: As ensembles combine multiple models, their decision-making process may become less interpretable, hindering clinical understanding.
2. **Computational complexity**: Ensembles may require more computational resources and time for training and prediction compared to individual models.
3. **Model diversity**: Ensuring sufficient diversity among base models is crucial for ensemble effectiveness. Ensuring diverse training data and model architectures is a challenge.

### 5.6.2 Addressing Uncertainty and Diversity in Ensemble Models

The diversity of base models in an ensemble is essential to prevent overfitting and improve generalization. Techniques such as bagging, boosting, and model stacking can enhance diversity. Additionally, handling prediction uncertainty is critical in clinical decision-making. Post-processing techniques, such as calibration and confidence estimation, can provide reliable uncertainty estimates. Overall, by addressing these challenges and harnessing the power of ensemble learning, we can enhance dis- ease diagnosis accuracy and improve patient care. The next section introduces the Teaching-Learning-Based Optimization algorithm and its potential application in disease diagnosis ensemble optimization.

## 5.7 PROPOSED MODEL WITH TEACHING-LEARNING-BASED OPTIMIZATION

In this section, we explore the TLBO algorithm, a nature-inspired optimization technique inspired by classroom teaching and learning processes. We have adapted the TLBO algorithm proposed by [6]. We provide an overview of TLBO, explain its algorithmic mechanics, and discuss its applications in the context of machine learning.

### 5.7.1 TLBO Overview

#### 5.7.1.1 Nature-Inspired Optimization Algorithms

Nature-inspired optimization algorithms are a class of computational techniques that mimic the natural processes observed in biological systems. These algorithms draw inspiration from natural phenomena such as evolution, swarm behavior, and ecological interactions to solve complex optimization problems. The overarching goal is to leverage the inherent efficiency and adaptability of nature to find optimal solutions in diverse domains.

#### 5.7.1.2 Introduction to TLBO

Teaching-learning-based optimization is one such nature-inspired optimization algorithm that was introduced by Rao et al. [6]. TLBO is based on the metaphor of teaching and learning in a classroom, where the better-performing students (solutions) share their knowledge with the weaker ones, collectively improving the overall learning outcome (optimization). TLBO is known for its simplicity, ease of implementation, and ability to handle continuous and discrete optimization problems.

### 5.7.2 TLBO Algorithm and Mechanics

#### 5.7.2.1 Teaching Phase and Learning Phase

The TLBO algorithm consists of two main phases: the teaching phase and the learning phase.

1. In the teaching phase, the best-performing solution (teacher) shares its knowledge with the other solutions (students) in the population.
2. In the learning phase, the students adjust their positions based on the teacher's knowledge, leading to a collective improvement of the entire population.

#### 5.7.2.2 TLBO Steps

The TLBO algorithm can be summarized in the following steps:

1. Initialize a population of solutions randomly.
2. Evaluate the fitness of each solution in the population.
3. Identify the best and worst solutions (teachers and students).
4. The teacher shares their knowledge (solution) with each student, updating their positions.
5. Recalculate the fitness of the updated population.
6. Repeat the teaching and learning phases until a termination criterion is met (e.g., maximum number of iterations or convergence).

The proposed model is shown in the Figure 5.1 and the steps of the proposed model are described in the following sections.

## 5.8 STEPS OF PROPOSED MODEL

1. **The TLBO algorithm**: The TLBO algorithm starts by creating multiple bags, each containing a random subset of the training data. These bags act as classrooms, and each classifier represents a student trying to learn from the

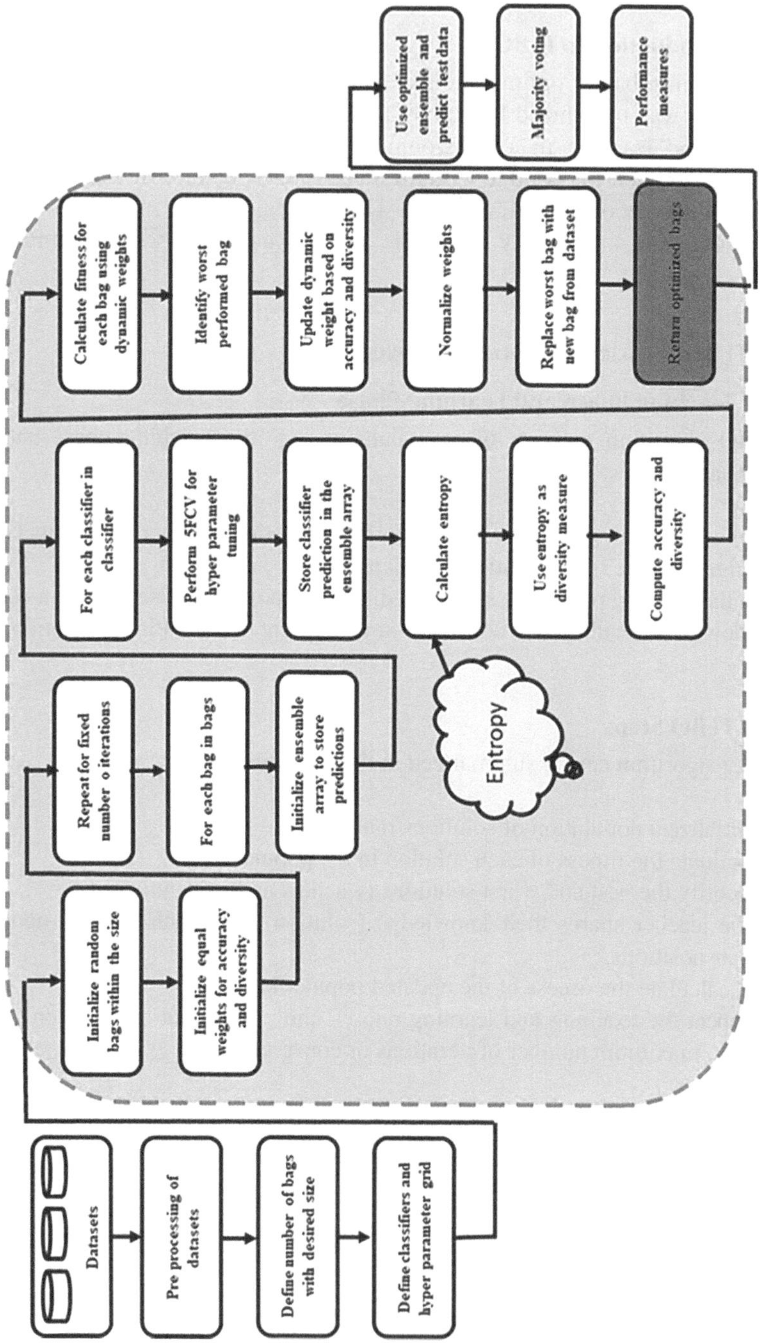


FIGURE 5.1 Proposed model.

data. The TLBO algorithm then uses a teaching strategy to guide the students (classifiers) toward better performance.

2. **Bag Initialization**: The TLBO algorithm begins by creating a fixed number of bags, each containing a random subset of the training data. This step ensures diversity among the bags, setting the stage for a diverse ensemble.
3. **Teaching and learning**: In each iteration, the TLBO algorithm evaluates the performance of each bag based on a weighted combination of accuracy and diversity. The diversity measure encourages classifiers to be different from each other, reducing the risk of redundant or correlated predictions.
4. **Dynamic weight update**: The algorithm dynamically updates the weights assigned to accuracy and diversity based on the relative performance of the classifiers. If the ensemble shows better accuracy than diversity, the weight for accuracy increases and vice versa. This dynamic weight update ensures that the ensemble converges towards an optimal balance between accuracy and diversity.
5. **Bag replacement**: The algorithm identifies the bag with the worst performance (worst bag) in each iteration and replaces it with a new randomly selected bag from the dataset. This step enables continuous exploration of different subsets of data and further enhances diversity in the ensemble.

In this section, we introduce the Dynamic Weighted Ensemble Approach, a novel technique that leverages the Teaching-Learning-Based Optimization (TLBO) algorithm to optimize the composition of an ensemble for disease diagnosis. This approach dynamically adjusts the classifier weights and ensemble size to improve diagnostic accuracy and robustness.

### 5.8.1 Ensemble Construction and Base Models

#### 5.8.1.1 Ensemble Construction

Ensemble learning involves combining multiple individual models (base models or classifiers) to create a more accurate and robust predictive model. The Dynamic Weighted Ensemble Approach builds an ensemble by selecting a diverse set of base classifiers, each of which is trained on a different subset of the data. The diversity among the base models is crucial for ensemble performance, as it allows the ensemble to capture different aspects of the underlying data distribution.

#### 5.8.1.2 Base Models

The base models used in the ensemble can vary, and they may belong to different algorithm families, such as DT, SVM, KNN, and LR. The choice of base models depends on the characteristics of the dataset and the nature of the disease diagnosis problem. By using a mix of classifiers, the ensemble can benefit from their complementary strengths and reduce the impact of individual model weaknesses.

### 5.8.2 Entropy-Based Diversity Measures

#### 5.8.2.1 Importance of Diversity in Ensembles

Diversity is a critical factor in ensemble learning, as it helps prevent overfitting and improves generalization performance. In the context of disease diagnosis, diversity among base classifiers is particularly relevant as it can capture different diagnostic patterns and enhance the ensemble's ability to handle a wide range of patient cases.

#### 5.8.2.2 Entropy as a Diversity Measure

Entropy is a widely used diversity measure in ensemble learning. It quantifies the uncertainty or disorder within a set of predictions made by different classifiers. In the Dynamic Weighted Ensemble Approach, entropy is used to measure the diversity among the base models' predictions for each patient sample. Higher entropy indicates higher disagreement among the classifiers, suggesting a more diverse set of predictions.

Entropy is a concept borrowed from information theory that serves as a diversity measure in various fields, including machine learning and ensemble learning. In the context of ensemble learning, entropy is used to quantify the diversity or dissimilarity of predictions made by different base models or classifiers within an ensemble.

To understand entropy as a diversity measure, let's consider its definition and properties:

#### 5.8.2.3 Definition of Entropy

Entropy is a measure of uncertainty or randomness in a probability distribution. In information theory, it is used to quantify the amount of information contained in a random variable. Mathematically, the entropy of a discrete random variable X with probability distribution P(X) is given by the following formula:

$$H(X) = -\sum P(x) \cdot \log_2 \left(P(x)\right) \tag{5.1}$$

where P(x) is the probability of occurrence of the value x, and the summation is taken over all possible values of X.

1. **Interpretation in ensemble learning**: In ensemble learning, each base model (e.g., decision tree, neural network, etc.) in the ensemble provides its predictions for a given instance in the dataset. These predictions can be seen as probability distributions over the class labels. The more diverse the predictions are among the base models, the higher the entropy, indicating greater uncertainty or lack of consensus among the models.
2. **High entropy vs. low entropy**:
    a. **High entropy**: When the predictions of the base models are diverse and spread out among different class labels for a given instance, the entropy is high. This indicates that the ensemble has high uncertainty about the correct class label for that instance.

   b. **Low entropy**: On the other hand, when the predictions are highly consistent and concentrated on a particular class label, the entropy is low. This suggests a high level of agreement and confidence among the base models.
   a. **Role in ensemble learning**: The use of entropy as a diversity measure in ensemble learning is essential for ensuring that the base models complement each other and cover different decision regions in the feature space. High diversity among the base models can lead to improved ensemble performance by reducing overfitting and enhancing generalization.
   b. **Calculating diversity using entropy**: To calculate diversity using entropy, the predictions of the base models for a specific instance are treated as probability distributions. The entropy is computed for each instance, and then the average or overall diversity across all instances in a bag (subset of the dataset) is calculated. This average entropy value represents the diversity of the bag, and lower values indicate higher agreement and similarity among the base models within the bag.
3. In summary, entropy is a diversity measure that quantifies the uncertainty and randomness in the predictions of different base models within an ensemble. It plays a crucial role in ensemble learning optimization algorithms, like the TLBO algorithm, to ensure that the ensemble benefits from the complementary strengths of its constituent models.

### 5.8.3 TLBO-Driven Optimization for Dynamic Ensemble

#### 5.8.3.1 TLBO Optimization of Ensemble Weights

The core of the Dynamic Weighted Ensemble Approach lies in using the TLBO algorithm to optimize the ensemble weights dynamically. TLBO drives the search for optimal ensemble weights by maximizing the ensemble's accuracy and diversity. During each iteration of TLBO, the algorithm updates the classifier weights based on their performance on the training data. This adaptability allows the ensemble to evolve and adapt to changes in the data distribution.

#### 5.8.3.2 Dynamic Ensemble Size Adjustment

In addition to adjusting classifier weights, TLBO also optimizes the ensemble's size. The number of base classifiers in the ensemble is a tunable parameter that can significantly impact its performance. TLBO dynamically determines the optimal ensemble size by evaluating the trade-off between accuracy and diversity. By selecting an appropriate ensemble size, the approach can achieve a balance between model complexity and generalization ability.

### 5.8.4 Fitness Function

The fitness function in the above code represents a measure of the overall performance of each bag (learner) in the Teaching-Learning-Based Optimization (TLBO) algorithm. The fitness function is used to evaluate the quality of each bag's solution (ensemble) and guide the optimization process toward finding better-performing solutions. In the context of the dynamic weighted ensemble approach for disease diagnosis, the fitness function is composed of two components: accuracy and diversity. Where:

1. **Accuracy weight** is a weight parameter that represents the importance of accuracy in the fitness function. It is updated dynamically during the optimization process, based on the bag's performance in each iteration.
2. **Accuracy** is the accuracy of the bag's ensemble predictions on the training data. It measures how well the ensemble correctly classifies instances.
3. **Diversity weight** is another weight parameter that indicates the significance of diversity in the fitness function. Like accuracy weight, it is updated dynamically during the optimization process.
4. **Diversity** is a measure of diversity among the predictions of the base classifiers within the bag's ensemble. It is calculated using the disagreement matrix, which quantifies the disagreement between the predictions of different classifiers in the ensemble. A lower value of diversity indicates that the classifiers' predictions are more similar, while a higher value indicates more disagreement.

The fitness function encourages the optimization algorithm to find a balance between accuracy and diversity in the bag's ensemble. By incorporating both accuracy and diversity in the fitness evaluation, the TLBO algorithm can explore different ensemble compositions and select the ones that not only perform well individually but also exhibit diversity in their predictions. This dynamic weighted ensemble approach aims to create an ensemble that is accurate and diverse, leading to improved disease diagnosis performance and robustness.

$$\text{Fitness}(f) = \text{mean}(\text{accuracies}) \times w_{\text{acc}} + \text{mean}(\text{diversities}) \times w_{\text{div}} \tag{5.2}$$

where mean (accuracies) is the mean accuracy of the bags in the ensemble; mean (diversities) is the mean diversity (entropy) of the bags in the ensemble; $w_{\text{acc}}$ is weight for accuracy; and $w_{\text{div}}$ is weight for diversity.

The entropy formula is given by:

$$\text{Entropy}(p) = -\sum_{i=1}^{n} p_i \log_2(p_i) \tag{5.3}$$

where $p$ is the probability distribution of classes, $p_i$ represents the probability of class $i$, and $n$ is the total number of classes.

### 5.8.5 Standard TLBO

TLBO is a population-based optimization algorithm inspired by the teaching and learning processes in a classroom. It was proposed to solve optimization problems, particularly continuous and global optimization problems. The TLBO algorithm generally comprises the following steps:

1. **Initialization**: Generate an initial population of candidate solutions (individuals) randomly within the problem domain.
2. **Objective function**: Define the objective function that needs to be optimized. The objective function evaluates the fitness of each candidate solution.
3. **Teaching phase**:
   a. Evaluate the fitness of each individual in the population using the objective function.
   b. Identify the best and worst solutions in the current population based on their fitness values.
4. **Learning phase**:
   a. For each student (individual) in the population, update their solution by learning from the teacher (best individual). This step mimics the learning process where students try to improve their solutions based on the teacher's performance.
   b. The new solution of the student is updated using a formula that takes into account the current solution and the teacher's solution.
5. **Population update**: Replace the worst solutions in the population with the newly updated solutions from the learning phase.
6. **Termination**: Repeat the teaching and learning phases until a termination condition is met (e.g., a maximum number of iterations is reached, or the convergence criterion is satisfied).

Algorithm 1 gives steps of the standard TLBO algorithm in which the teaching phase and learning phase explain how the fitness is computed and also explained in the algorithm.

---

**Algorithm 1:** Teaching-Learning-Based Optimization (TLBO)

---

```
Input : population size, max iterations, termination criterion
Output: best solution

Initialize the population randomly;
Evaluate the fitness of each solution;

for iteration = 1 to max iterations do
    best solution → None;
    worst solution → None;
    // Identify the best and worst solutions (teachers and students)
    for each solution in population do
        if best solution is None or fitness(solution) > fitness(best solution)
          then
            best solution → solution;
        end
```

```
        if worst solution is None or fitness(solution) < fitness(worst solution)
          then
            worst solution → solution;
        end
    end
    // Teaching Phase
    for each student in population do
        if student is not equal to best solution then
            teacher → best solution;
        end
        else
            teacher → randomly˙select˙teacher˙except(student,
              best˙solution);
        end
        // Update student's position based on the teacher's knowledge
        for each variable in student do
            teaching mean → (teacher.variable + student.variable) / 2;
            random number → random˙uniform˙between(0, 1);
            student.variable → student.variable + random˙number *
            (teacher.variable - teaching˙mean);
        end
        // Ensure the student's position remains within the feasible bounds
    end
    // Recalculate fitness of the updated population
    Evaluate the fitness of each solution;

    // Check termination criterion
    if termination˙criterion˙met() then
        break;
    end
end

return best˙solution;
```

### 5.8.6 Adaptive TLBO for Ensemble Approach

**Algorithm 2:** Teaching-Learning-Based Optimization for Adaptive Ensemble Optimization (TLBO-AEO)

**Data:** Dataset, Classifiers, no_of_bags, min_bag_ size, max_bag_size, no_of_iterations

**Output:** Optimal_bags, Worst_bag_accuracies, Worst_bag_diversities, Worst_bag_fitness

Randomly initialize bags *bags* with *num*$_b$*ags*; Initialize *w_acc* = 0.5 and *w_div* = 0.5;
Initialize tracking lists: *worst˙bag˙accuracies*, *worst_bag_diversities*, *worst_bag_f itnesses*;
**for** *iteration in range(num˙iterations)* **do**
  Initialize *accuracies* and *diversities*;
  **for** *bag in bags* **do**
    Split *data* into *X _train_bag* and *y_train_bag* based on *bag*;
    Initialize *ensemble˙preds* and *entropies*;
    **for** (*name, cl f*) *in classi f iers* **do**
      Train *model* using 5-fold cross-validation on *X _train_bag* and *y_train_bag* with hyperparameter grid *cl f* [*param_grid*];
      Predict *preds* on *X _train_bag*;
      Update *ensemble_preds* and calculate entropy for classifier's predictions;
    Calculate diversity as the average entropy of classifiers' predictions;
    Calculate accuracy using majority voting;
    Append *accuracy* and *diversity* to *accuracies* and *diversities*;
  Calculate *f itness* f using Eq. 5.2 for each bag using dynamic weights;
  Identify the worst bag with the lowest fitness;
  Record the worst bag's accuracy, diversity, and fitness;
  Update dynamic weights for accuracy and diversity based on the ensemble's performance;
  Normalize the weights to sum up to 1;
  Replace the worst bag with a new bag randomly sampled from *data*;
  Update *bags*;
  Append worst bag accuracy, diversity, and fitness to tracking lists;

**return** *optimal_bags*, *worst_bag_accuracies*, *worst_bag_diversities*, *worst_bag_f itnesses*;

The proposed model is explained by Algorithm 2, in which fitness weights are updated adaptively the fitness of the best and worst bag is computed, and each iteration of the bag adjusts the components and computes the fitness of the bag with unique fitness functions.

Ensemble learning techniques have been widely utilized to improve the performance and robustness of machine learning models. In this study, we proposed a novel

The proposed model is explained by Algorithm 2, in which fitness weights are updated, the fitness of the best and worst bag is computed, and each iteration of the bag adjusts the components and computes the fitness of the bag with unique fitness functions.

Ensemble learning techniques have been widely utilized to improve the performance and robustness of machine learning models. In this study, we proposed a novel

TLBO algorithm to dynamically select and combine classifiers within an ensemble for enhanced predictive accuracy and diversity. The proposed approach aims to address the challenge of selecting an optimal ensemble from a diverse set of classifiers, each with its unique hyperparameters. Ensemble learning has proven to be a powerful technique for improving model accuracy and generalization. The key idea behind ensemble learning is to combine predictions from multiple models to achieve better results than any single model. While there are various methods for building ensembles, selecting an optimal ensemble from a diverse pool of classifiers remains a challenging task. The TLBO algorithm, inspired by the teaching-learning process in a classroom, is a unique approach that dynamically adapts ensemble selection and promotes diversity among the base classifiers. The proposed model is shown in the Figure 5.1.

## 5.9 CASE STUDY: COMPUTING ENTROPY IN THE DYNAMIC WEIGHTED ENSEMBLE APPROACH

Let's consider a case study to demonstrate how to compute entropy in the Dynamic Weighted Ensemble Approach for disease diagnosis. In this case study, we have an ensemble consisting of four base classifiers (KNN, DT, SVM, and LR). The ensemble is trained on a dataset of patients with binary labels (healthy or diseased).

1. **Step 1**: **Ensemble Predictions**. After training the ensemble on the dataset, we obtain the predictions of each base classifier for a specific patient sample. Let's assume the predictions for the patient sample are as follows: K- Nearest Neighbors: Predicts 'Healthy'; Decision Tree: Predicts 'Diseased'; Support Vector Machine: Predicts 'Healthy'
2. **Step 2**: **Calculating Probabilities**. Next, we calculate the probability distribution of class predictions for the patient sample. Since the ensemble consists of three classifiers, there are two classes: 'Healthy' and 'Diseased.' We count the occurrences of each class prediction and divide by the total number of classifiers (3) to get the probabilities:

$$Probability\,of\,"Healthy"\,class: p_{Healthy} = \frac{2}{3} \tag{5.4}$$

$$Probability\,of\,"Diseased"\,class: p_{Diseased} = \frac{1}{3} \tag{5.5}$$

3. **Step 3**: Now, we can calculate the entropy for the patient sample using the probabilities obtained in Step 2. The entropy formula is given by Equation (5.3).

Substituting the probabilities, we get:

$$\begin{aligned}\text{Entropy} &= -\left(\frac{2}{3}\log_2\left(\frac{2}{3}\right)+\frac{1}{3}\log_2\left(\frac{1}{3}\right)\right)\\ &= -\left(\frac{2}{3}\times(-0.58496)+\frac{1}{3}\times(1.58496)\right)\\ &= -(-0.38997+0.52832)\\ &= 0.13835\end{aligned}$$

Using the base-2 logarithm, the entropy of the ensemble for the given patient sample is calculated to be 0.13835. This value represents the level of uncertainty or disorder in the ensemble's predictions for the patient sample, reflecting the diversity among the base classifiers' opinions.

### 5.9.1 Applications of TLBO in Machine Learning

#### 5.9.1.1 Overview of TLBO's Applications in Different Domains

The TLBO algorithm has found applications in various domains, including engineering optimization, data mining, image processing, and machine learning. Its ability to handle continuous and discrete optimization problems, combined with its simplicity, has made TLBO an attractive choice for solving complex real-world optimization tasks.

### 5.9.2 TLBO in Ensemble Learning and Model Optimization

In the context of machine learning, TLBO has been utilized for ensemble learning and model optimization. By incorporating TLBO into ensemble learning, it becomes possible to dynamically optimize the ensemble's performance by adjusting the classifier weights and ensemble size. TLBO can be leveraged to enhance the diversity of base classifiers, adaptively adjust their contributions, and improve the overall performance of the ensemble system. By leveraging TLBO's teaching and learning mechanisms, the proposed approach aims to create an ensemble system that optimally combines diverse classifiers for disease diagnosis, leading to improved accuracy and robustness. The subsequent section delves into the details of the dynamic weighted ensemble approach and its integration with TLBO for disease diagnosis optimization.

## 5.10 EXPERIMENTAL SETUP AND RESULTS

In this experiment, we utilized the HP Compaq Intel® Core™ i7-1065G7 CPU paired with 8 GB RAM to conduct our research. Our proposed methodology and results analysis were meticulously carried out using Python, along with the widely acclaimed sklearn library.

### 5.10.1 Dataset Description

**Pima Indian Dataset:**

The Pima Indian dataset is widely used for diabetes classification tasks. It comprises 768 instances, each representing medical data for a female patient of Pima Indian heritage. The dataset contains eight features, including glucose concentration, blood pressure, and body mass index, along with the patient's age and pregnancy history. The goal is to predict whether a patient has diabetes (Positive class) or not (Negative class) based on the provided features. Due to its relevance in diabetes research, this dataset has been extensively used to develop and evaluate machine-learning algorithms for disease diagnosis and predictive modeling.

**Statlog Heart Dataset:**

The Statlog Heart dataset focuses on heart disease diagnosis and consists of 270 instances. Each instance represents medical data for a patient, including 13 features such as age, chest pain type, cholesterol levels, and resting electrocardiogram results. The target variable is binary, indicating the presence (Present class) or absence (Absent class) of heart disease in the patient. Researchers and clinicians often utilize this dataset to develop and assess machine learning models for early detection and diagnosis of heart-related conditions, contributing to cardiovascular health assessment and risk prediction.

**Wilson Breast Cancer Dataset:**

The Wilson Breast Cancer dataset focuses on breast cancer diagnosis and consists of 699 instances. Each instance represents medical data for a patient, including nine features like tumor size, clump thickness, and mitoses count. The dataset's target variable is binary, indicating whether the tumor is malignant (Malignant class) or benign (Benign class). This dataset has been widely used to develop machine learning models for breast cancer detection, providing insights into the classification of breast tumors and assisting clinicians in making informed decisions regarding diagnosis and treatment planning.

Table 5.1 provides an overview of all the data sets used in the study, while this preprocessing step ensures that the data is appropriately prepared for building the dynamic weighted ensemble model.

### 5.10.2 Evaluation Metrics

All the evaluation metrics used in this are explained in [5, 15].

It is essential to consider these diverse metrics to gain a comprehensive understanding of the model's performance across different evaluation aspects. By doing so, we can effectively and reliably evaluate the model's predictive capabilities and draw meaningful conclusions from the experimental results.

By considering this comprehensive set of metrics, the evaluation process provides a holistic understanding of the proposed model's performance across different aspects of disease diagnosis.

**TABLE 5.1**
**Datasets Used in the Proposed Study**

| Dataset | Description | Instances | Features | Class Labels |
|---|---|---|---|---|
| Pima Indian | Diabetes classification | 768 | 8 | 2 (Positive/ Negative) |
| Statlog Heart | Heart disease diagnosis | 270 | 13 | 2 (Present/Absent) |
| Wilson Breast Cancer | Breast cancer diagnosis | 699 | 9 | 2 (Malignant/ Benign) |

**TABLE 5.2**
**Confusion Matrix**

| | | Predicted | |
|---|---|---|---|
| | | **Diseased** | **Healthy** |
| **Actual** | **Diseased** | TP | FN |
| | **Healthy** | FP | TN |

The performance of the proposed model is assessed using a range of evaluation metrics such as the confusion matrix, which is shown in Table 5.2, each offering valuable insights into the model's predictive capabilities for disease diagnosis. The metrics are defined as follows:

$$\text{Accuracy} = \frac{TP + TN}{TP + TN + FP + FN} \tag{5.10}$$

$$\text{Specificity} = \frac{TN}{TN + FP} \tag{5.11}$$

$$\text{G-measure} = \sqrt{\text{Specificity} \times \text{Sensitivity}} \tag{5.12}$$

$$\text{Precision} = \frac{TP}{TP + FP} \tag{5.13}$$

$$\text{F1-score} = 2 \times \frac{\text{Precision} \times \text{Recall}}{\text{Precision} + \text{Recall}} \tag{5.14}$$

$$\text{False Positive Rate}\left(\text{FPR}\right) = \frac{FP}{FP + TN} \tag{5.15}$$

$$\text{Sensitivity}\left(\text{Recall}\right) \text{ or True Positive Rate } \left(\text{TPR}\right) = \frac{TP}{TP+FN} \tag{5.16}$$

Whereas the notation used in the evaluation includes the following components:

TP (True Positives) represents the cases that the classifier correctly identifies as disease positive.
TN (True Negatives) represents the cases that the classifier correctly identifies as disease negative.
FP (False Positives) represents the cases that are incorrectly classified as disease positive by the classifier.
FN (False Negatives) represents the cases that are incorrectly classified as disease negative by the classifier.

In addition to the ROC curve, the Area Under the ROC curve (AUC) score provides a quantitative measure of the model's ability to effectively differentiate between the disease classes. The AUC score offers a comprehensive evaluation of the model's predictive performance, taking into account its sensitivity and specificity.

By incorporating these essential components in the evaluation process, we can gain valuable insights into the model's capacity to accurately classify disease instances, thereby enabling informed decision-making and enhancing the overall reliability of the model's predictions.

### 5.10.3 Experimental Design and Methodology

The experimental design and methodology of the proposed model are as follows:

1. **Dataset selection**: The first step in the experimental design is to select the disease datasets for evaluation. In this case, three datasets are chosen: the Pima Indian Diabetes dataset (PID), Statlog Heart Data (SHD), and the Wisconsin Breast Cancer dataset (WBC). Each dataset contains medical data related to specific diseases, and the goal is to develop a dynamic weighted ensemble model for disease diagnosis.
2. **Data pre-processing**: Data pre-processing is a crucial phase performed on the disease datasets before constructing the ensemble model. The objective is to enhance data quality and ensure its suitability for effective modeling.

   The following pre-processing steps are applied to achieve these goals
   a. **Replacing zero values**: Zero values in the dataset are replaced with the median value of the respective feature. This approach helps to handle missing or incomplete data and prevents any undue influence of outliers.
   b. **Identifying numerical and binary columns**: The dataset is carefully examined to identify columns containing numerical and binary data. This differentiation is essential as it guides specific pre-processing techniques for each data type.

c. **Label encoding for binary columns**: For binary columns, a label encoding technique is applied to convert categorical binary variables into numerical form. This facilitates ease of computation and allows the model to process the data effectively.
d. **Duplicating multivalue columns**: Certain columns with multivalued attributes may need to be duplicated or transformed using one-hot encoding. This step ensures that categorical variables are appropriately represented for the ensemble model.
e. **Scaling numerical features**: To bring numerical features to a consistent scale, standard scaling is performed. This process standardizes the features, making them comparable and avoiding any undue biases during the modeling process.
f. **Merging scaled values for numerical columns**: After scaling, the numerical features are merged back into the dataset to form a unified and pre-processed dataset suitable for building the ensemble model.

These data pre-processing steps are essential to ensure that the data used for the ensemble model is of high quality, consistent, and devoid of any inconsistencies that could affect the model's predictive performance. By carefully handling missing values, encoding categorical data, and standardizing numerical features, the ensemble model can effectively leverage the pre-processed dataset to make accurate and reliable predictions related to the disease classification task.

3. **Teaching-learning-based optimization (TLBO)**: The proposed ensemble model utilizes the TLBO algorithm to optimize the ensemble's composition dynamically. TLBO is a nature-inspired optimization algorithm that simulates the teaching and learning process among a population of learners. It involves random initialization of the learners (bags), evaluation of fitness, and iterative updates based on the performance of the bags.
4. **Dynamic weighted ensemble construction**: During the TLBO-driven optimization process, the algorithm updates the ensemble's weights dynamically based on the bag's performance. The weights are adjusted according to the accuracy and diversity of the bags, allowing the ensemble to adapt and learn from the best-performing bags over iterations.
5. **Model evaluation**: After obtaining the optimal ensemble composition, the model is evaluated using various performance metrics, including accuracy, sensitivity, specificity, G-measure, precision, recall, and F1-score. These metrics are derived from the confusion matrix, which summarizes the model's predictions.
6. **Comparison with baseline methods**: The performance of the proposed dynamic weighted ensemble model is compared against baseline methods, which may include other traditional ensemble techniques or individual classifiers. This comparison allows for assessing the effectiveness of the proposed approach in disease diagnosis.
7. **Statistical analysis**: Statistical tests may be applied to validate the significance of the performance improvements achieved by the proposed model

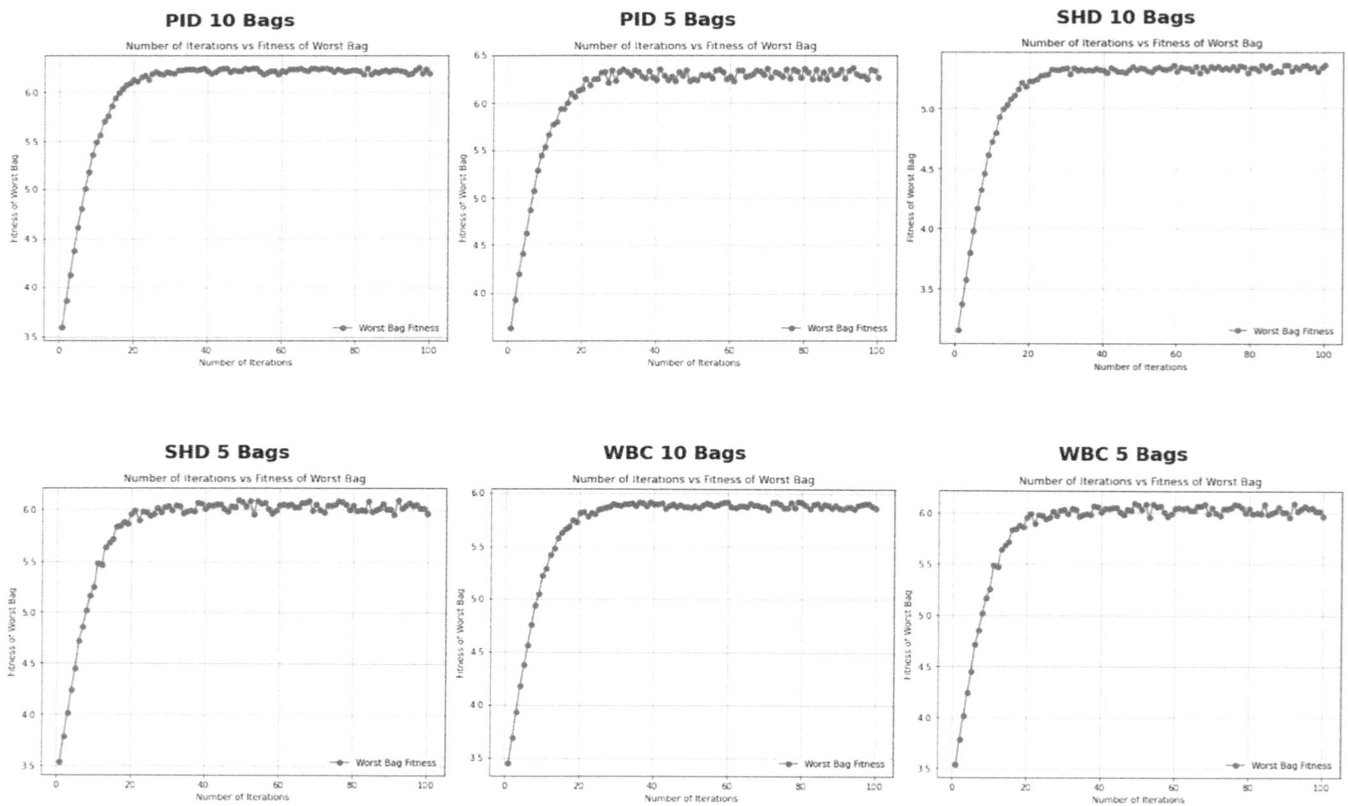


**FIGURE 5.2** Convergence plots of the proposed model on PID, SHD, and WBC (Fitness vs No of iterations).

compared to baseline methods. Techniques like t-tests or ANOVA can be used to determine the statistical significance of the results.

8. **Cross-validation**: To ensure the robustness of the model and reduce over-Dynamic Weighted Ensemble Framework fitting, k-fold cross-validation is often employed during training and evaluation. Cross-validation involves partitioning the dataset into k subsets, using k-1 subsets for training, and one subset for validation in each iteration.
9. **Practical implications and interpretability**: The study also explores the practical implications of the proposed dynamic ensemble model in clinical settings. The interpretability of the model's predictions and its integration with decision support systems are discussed to understand its potential real-world applications.

## 5.11 RESULTS ANALYSIS

In the proposed model all three disease datasets are preprocessed and preprocessed datasets are split into training and testing sets with 80% and 20%, respectively. The 80% of training data sets undergo TLBO-based optimization, whereas the 20% are not used in the training process. Training and testing phases are explained step-by-step as follows.

### 5.11.1 Training and Testing Phase of Proposed Model

1. **Training phase**:
   a. The TLBO optimization algorithm is applied to find the optimal bags (subsets of the training data) and classifiers' ensemble weights based on accuracy and diversity.

**TABLE 5.3**
**5FCV Performance of Various Classifiers before Applying Proposed Model**

| Dataset | Classifier | Accuracy | AUC | Sensitivity | Specificity |
|---|---|---|---|---|---|
| | LR | 0.765 | 0.795 | 0.784 | 0.765 |
| | KNN | 0.834 | 0.842 | 0.857 | 0.865 |
| PID | SVM | 0.864 | 0.854 | 0.842 | 0.856 |
| | DT | 0.845 | 0.824 | 0.896 | 0.824 |
| | LR | 0.745 | 0.789 | 0.784 | 0.732 |
| | KNN | 0.832 | 0.857 | 0.865 | 0.847 |
| WBC | SVM | 0.887 | 0.865 | 0.872 | 0.833 |
| | DT | 0.842 | 0.859 | 0.822 | 0.866 |
| | LR | 0.772 | 0.785 | 0.803 | 0.823 |
| | KNN | 0.851 | 0.844 | 0.836 | 0.872 |
| SHD | SVM | 0.862 | 0.854 | 0.822 | 0.866 |
| | DT | 0.824 | 0.856 | 0.874 | 0.869 |

**TABLE 5.4**
**Hyper Parameters of Various Classifiers over Various Datasets**

| Dataset | LR | KNN | SVM | DT |
|---|---|---|---|---|
| PID | C=0.01 | #neighbors = 11 | C =50<br>gamma =0.001<br>kernel = RBF | SC = Gini<br>Depth =6 |
| SHD | C=0.01 | #neighbors = 5 | C =100<br>gamma =0.001<br>kernel = RBF | SC = Gini<br>Depth =5 |
| WBC | C=0.001 | #neighbors = 11 | C =50<br>gamma =0.01<br>kernel = RBF | SC = Gini<br>Depth =6 |
| C | Regularization Parameter | gamma | RBF kernel coefficient | |
| SC | Splitting Criteria | Depth | Maximum depth of DT | |
| RBF | Radial Basis Function | | | |

**TABLE 5.5**
**Worst Bag Optimization Using TLBO with 10 Bags**

| Dataset | Iteration | Worst bag accuracy | Worst bag diversity | Worst bag fitness |
|---|---|---|---|---|
| PID | 0 | 0.942 | 5.95 | 5.62 |
| | 20 | 0.968 | 6.52 | 6.12 |
| | 40 | 0.971 | 6.34 | 6.22 |
| | 60 | 0.964 | 6.28 | 6.21 |
| | 80 | 0.981 | 6.33 | 6.22 |
| | 100 | 0.982 | 6.04 | 6.19 |
| WBC | 0 | 0.990 | 6.01 | 5.52 |
| | 20 | 0.998 | 6.32 | 5.81 |
| | 40 | 0.993 | 6.12 | 5.89 |
| | 60 | 0.996 | 6.22 | 5.91 |
| | 80 | 0.989 | 6.30 | 5.91 |
| | 100 | 0.994 | 5.78 | 5.86 |
| SHD | 0 | 0.921 | 5.03 | 5.11 |
| | 20 | 0.945 | 5.18 | 5.23 |
| | 40 | 0.935 | 5.13 | 5.32 |
| | 60 | 0.993 | 5.03 | 5.31 |
| | 80 | 0.927 | 5.32 | 5.34 |
| | 100 | 0.969 | 5.56 | 5.36 |

**TABLE 5.6**
**Worst Bag Optimization Using TLBO with 5 Bags**

| Dataset | Iteration | Worst bag accuracy | Worst bag diversity | Worst bag fitness |
|---|---|---|---|---|
| PID | 0 | 0.942 | 5.95 | 5.62 |
| | 20 | 0.975 | 6.05 | 6.14 |
| | 40 | 0.933 | 5.94 | 6.23 |
| | 60 | 0.959 | 6.16 | 6.28 |
| | 80 | 0.974 | 6.56 | 6.36 |
| | 100 | 0.956 | 6.09 | 6.26 |
| WBC | 0 | 0.935 | 5.85 | 5.92 |
| | 20 | 0.994 | 6.20 | 5.96 |
| | 40 | 0.992 | 5.92 | 6.01 |
| | 60 | 0.995 | 6.04 | 6.04 |
| | 80 | 0.984 | 6.06 | 6.04 |
| | 100 | 0.996 | 5.69 | 5.97 |
| SHD | 0 | 0.935 | 5.23 | 5.65 |
| | 20 | 0.942 | 5.14 | 5.16 |
| | 40 | 0.948 | 5.24 | 5.28 |
| | 60 | 0.949 | 5.31 | 5.29 |
| | 80 | 0.950 | 5.43 | 5.31 |
| | 100 | 0.952 | 5.26 | 5.28 |

**TABLE 5.7**
**Proposed Model Performance on PID, WBC, and SHD Datasets with 10 Bags**

| Dataset | Accuracy | AUC | Precision | Recall | F1 Score | G-Measure |
|---|---|---|---|---|---|---|
| PID | 0.909 | 0.905 | 0.859 | 0.890 | 0.875 | 0.904 |
| WBC | 0.991 | 0.988 | 0.99 | 0.976 | 0.988 | 0.988 |
| SHD | 0.907 | 0.889 | 0.944 | 0.809 | 0.871 | 0.885 |

**TABLE 5.8**
**Proposed Model Performance on PID, WBC, and SHD Datasets with 5 Bags**

| Dataset | Accuracy | AUC | Precision | Recall | F1 Score | G-Measure |
|---|---|---|---|---|---|---|
| PID | 0.922 | 0.911 | 0.905 | 0.872 | 0.888 | 0.910 |
| WBC | 0.982 | 0.981 | 0.976 | 0.976 | 0.976 | 0.981 |
| SHD | 0.907 | 0.906 | 0.863 | 0.904 | 0.883 | 0.906 |

   b. During the TLBO optimization, bags are randomly initialized, and classifiers are trained using the hyperparameter grids and cross-validation on the bags.
   c. The TLBO optimization process iteratively replaces the worst- performing bag with a new randomly sampled bag from the training data.
2. **Testing phase**:
   a. After the TLBO optimization is completed and the optimal bags are identified, the ensemble predictions are made on the testing data using the trained classifiers and the optimal weights obtained during the optimization.
   b. The ensemble predictions are calculated by majority voting, where each classifier's prediction contributes one vote, and the final prediction is the one with the most votes.
   c. The evaluation metrics, such as accuracy, AUC, sensitivity, specificity, precision, F1 score, and G-measure, are then calculated based on the ensemble predictions and compared with the true labels in the testing data.
   d. It's important to note that the testing phase is separate from the TLBO optimization process. The TLBO optimization is only applied during the training phase to find the optimal ensemble weights and subsets of the training data (bags). Once the optimization is complete, the model is fixed, and no further training occurs.

So, in summary, after the TLBO optimization during the training phase, the testing phase involves using the optimized ensemble of classifiers to predict the labels on the testing data and evaluate the model's performance using various evaluation metrics.

## 5.12 K-FOLD CROSS VALIDATION IN PROPOSED MODEL

In the above approach, K-Fold Cross-Validation [16] is used during the training phase to evaluate the performance of each bag (a subset of data) for each classifier in the ensemble. K-Fold Cross-Validation is a common technique to assess the generalization ability of a machine learning model and helps to reduce the risk of overfitting. Here's how K-Fold Cross-Validation is applied in the training phase of the proposed approach (here k=5):

1. **K-Fold Cross-Validation for individual classifiers**:
   a. For each bag during the training phase, the dataset is split into K (commonly set to 5) equally sized folds. One of the folds is used as the validation set, while the remaining K-1 folds are used as the training set.
   b. The training set is used to fine-tune the classifier's hyperparameters, while the validation set is used to assess them. Each fold serves as the validation set once during the K-fold iteration of this process. The classifier's performance statistic for that specific bag is its average performance (for example, accuracy) over the K runs.

2. **Ensemble creation and diversity calculation**:
   a. After training each classifier using K-Fold Cross-Validation on each bag, the ensemble's performance on a bag is evaluated based on the average performance of the individual classifiers trained on that bag.
   b. In addition to accuracy, the diversity of the ensemble is also calculated. Diversity is measured by calculating the entropy of the class predictions made by each classifier on the training set of the bag.
   c. The diversity is used to ensure that the classifiers in the ensemble are not highly correlated, as diverse classifiers tend to lead to better ensemble performance.
      i. **Fitness calculation**:
         A. The performance of a bag in the ensemble is quantified by a fitness value, which is calculated based on the dynamic weights for accuracy and diversity.
         B. The fitness of a bag is defined as the weighted sum of accuracy and diversity, where the weights are dynamically adjusted during the optimization process.
         C. The goal of the TLBO algorithm is to find the bags that contribute the most to the overall performance of the ensemble, as measured by the fitness value.
      ii. **Bag replacement and optimization**:
         A. In each iteration of the TLBO algorithm, the bag with the worst fitness (lowest performance) is identified.
         B. The bag with the worst performance is replaced by a new bag randomly sampled from the entire dataset, and the optimization process continues.
         C. This bag replacement and optimization procedure continues for a specified number of iterations to improve the overall ensemble's performance.

In summary, K-Fold Cross-Validation is used to train and evaluate individual classifiers on different subsets of the data (bags) during the training phase. The performance of each bag is assessed using K-Fold Cross-Validation, and the diversity of the ensemble is calculated to ensure the classifiers are diverse. The TLBO algorithm uses the fitness value, which incorporates both accuracy and diversity, to dynamically optimize the ensemble by iteratively replacing the worst-performing bags. This iterative optimization process aims to improve the overall performance and robustness of the ensemble.

### 5.12.1 Majority Voting

In the provided approach using the TLBO algorithm for ensemble learning, the final prediction is made using majority voting. Let's go through the steps of how majority voting is applied in this specific approach:

1. **Ensemble training**: The ensemble consists of multiple base classifiers, including LR, KNN, SVM, and DT. Each of these classifiers is trained on a randomly selected bag of training data.

2. **Prediction generation**: After training the base classifiers on their respective bags, they are used to make predictions on the training instances within their bags. For each instance in a bag, all the classifiers in the ensemble provide a prediction.
3. **Voting**: The predictions made by the classifiers within each bag are collected. The predictions can be binary (0 or 1) for binary classification or multiclass labels for a multiclass problem.
4. **Majority decision**: To make the final prediction for each instance in a bag, majority voting is applied. In majority voting, the class that appears most frequently in the predictions of the classifiers within the bag is selected as the final prediction for that instance. For example, suppose the predictions made by the classifiers in a bag are as follows:

   Classifier 1: Class 1 Classifier 2: Class 0 Classifier 3: Class 1 Classifier 4: Class 1
   In this case, Class 1 appears three times (out of four predictions) and Class 0 appears once. Therefore, the final prediction for this instance in the bag will be Class 1, as it has the majority of votes.

5. **Ensemble prediction**: The above majority voting process is performed for each instance in each bag, resulting in a set of ensemble predictions for the entire training dataset.
6. **Testing prediction**: For the testing phase, the trained classifiers in the ensemble are used to make predictions on the unseen test data.
7. **Majority voting on testing data**: Similar to the training phase, majority voting is applied to the predictions made by the ensemble members for each instance in the test data. The class with the majority of votes across the classifiers is selected as the final prediction for each instance in the test data.

By the above experimental design and methodology, the study aims to demonstrate the effectiveness and potential impact of the proposed dynamic weighted ensemble approach in disease diagnosis and improve the overall accuracy and reliability of disease classification systems.

Our approach first evaluated the individual classifier performance on training data before applying the proposed model and the results are shown in Table 5.3. Further to improve the predictive model performance hyperparameter optimization uses grid search and hyperparameter values are tabulated, as shown in Table 5.4. Hyperparameters were optimized for each classifier. Further, to improve the performance we used the proposed TLBO with a fixed number of bags but bag size dynamically varies between half of the training data to the entire training data. This dynamic bag size maintains diversity and improves the generalization of model performance.

In this study a novel fitness function is introduced that consists of accuracy and diversity (entropy) and it adapts the weights of both measures within the TLBO optimization process. Here training data is split into bags and every bag undergoes an optimization process with provided classifiers such as LR, KNN, DT, and SVM.

All these classifiers compute accuracy and diversity and the mean of accuracy and diversity used in the fitness of the bag with dynamic weights based on accuracy and diversity measures. Each time, the best and worst bags are identified based on their fitness values. The samples in the bag with the lowest fitness are then replaced with new samples of the same size from the dataset. This process continues for a fixed number of iterations, during which the fitness of the worst bag gradually improves due to the introduction of diverse data samples. Once the termination conditions are satisfied, the optimal set of bags is generated. This optimal bag ensemble configuration is then used for testing, and finally, predictions are obtained on the test data.

We evaluated the performance of the proposed model on the PID, WBC, and SHD datasets using several bag sizes (10 and 5) over 100 iterations. The results were analyzed at every 20-iteration interval. The results were tabulated and are shown in Tables 5.5 and5.6, and a summary of the results with 10 bags and 5 bags are also shown in Tables 5.7 and 5.8.

Our study evaluated the robustness of the proposed model with the performance growth of the worst bag with several iterations and convergence. Performance on various datasets with 10 bags and 5 bags were plotted and are shown in Figure 5.2. From Figure 5.2, we can observe that the proposed model converges more effectively with 10 bags compared to 5 bags on the PID, SHD, and WBC datasets. This comparative performance is clearly illustrated in Figure 5.2.

### 5.12.2 Statistical Paired T-test

To perform statistical analysis using paired t-tests on the four datasets (PID, SHD, and WBC), we undertook the following steps. The results were tabulated and are shown in Table 5.9.

1. **Null and alternative hypotheses**: Define the null and alternative hypotheses for the paired t-tests. For example:
   a. **Null hypothesis (H0)**: There is no significant difference in the performance of the optimized ensemble compared to the individual classifiers or baseline ensemble methods.
   b. **Alternative hypothesis (HA)**: There is a significant difference in the performance of the optimized ensemble compared to the individual classifiers or baseline ensemble methods.
2. **Select performance metric**: Choose a specific performance metric to compare across the datasets. This could be accuracy, AUC, precision, recall, or F1-measure. Ensure that the chosen metric is suitable for the problem at hand.
3. **Data preparation**: Calculate the performance metric for each dataset using the optimized ensemble, individual classifiers, and baseline ensemble methods. Obtain a set of performance values for each method and dataset.
4. **Paired t-test**: Perform a paired t-test on the performance metric for each dataset to assess the statistical significance of the differences between

the methods. The paired t-test compares the means of two paired samples, considering the dependence between them.

5. **Statistical software or libraries**: Utilize statistical software or Python libraries (such as SciPy or stats models) to conduct the paired t-test. These libraries provide functions to calculate the t-value, degrees of freedom, and p-value.
6. **Calculate t-value and p-value**: Calculate the t-value and p-value using the paired t-test function or module in the statistical software or Python libraries. The t-value represents the magnitude of the difference between the means of the paired samples, while the p-value indicates the probability of obtaining the observed difference if the null hypothesis is true.
7. **Set significance level**: Choose a significance level (alpha) to determine the threshold for rejecting the null hypothesis. Commonly used significance levels are 0.05.
8. **Interpretation**: Compare the calculated p-value with the chosen significance level. If the p-value is less than the significance level, reject the null hypothesis and conclude that there is a significant difference in performance between the methods. If the p-value is greater than the significance level, fail to reject the null hypothesis and conclude that there is no significant difference.
9. **Repeat for each dataset**: Repeat the paired t-test analysis for each dataset, considering the specific performance metric chosen in step 2.
10. **Results and conclusion of t-test**: Summarize the results of the paired t-tests for each dataset. Report the calculated t-values, degrees of freedom, p-values, and the decision regarding the null hypothesis. Provide a conclusion on whether the optimized ensemble exhibits a statistically significant difference in performance compared to the individual classifiers or baseline ensemble methods for each dataset.

By conducting paired t-tests, you can assess the statistical significance of the performance differences between the optimized ensemble and the other methods on the four datasets. This analysis provides valuable insights into the effectiveness of the proposed approach and its superiority, if applicable, in terms of the chosen performance metric.

Finally, results are compared with the state-of-the-art (SOTA) ensemble and non-ensemble models, and comparative results are tabulated and shown in Table 5.10 and Table 5.11 and best results are highlighted. From the comparison with the SOTA ensemble, our proposed model's performance is superior in terms of Accuracy, AUC, Sensitivity, and Specificity. In comparison with the non-ensemble model, the proposed model's performance is superior in terms of Accuracy, AUC, Sensitivity, Precision, and F1 score. In the majority of the cases with 10 bags the proposed model's performance is more effective than with 5 bags.

**TABLE 5.9**
**Statical Analysis of the Proposed Model with Baseline Models on WBC, PID, and SHD**

| Dataset | proposed vs KNN | proposed vs LR | proposed vs DT | proposed vs SVM |
|---|---|---|---|---|
| WBC | 0.0010 | 0.024 | 0.003 | 0.017 |
| PID | 0.036 | 0.034 | 0.017 | 0.014 |
| SHD | 0.04 | 0.029 | 0.0038 | 0.001 |

## 5.13 PRACTICAL IMPLICATIONS AND FUTURE DIRECTIONS

In this final section, we discuss the practical implications of the Dynamic Weighted Ensemble Approach for disease diagnosis and explore potential future directions for advancing the technique.

### 5.13.1 Clinical Application and Interoperability

#### 5.13.1.1 Real-world Clinical Applications

The Dynamic Weighted Ensemble Approach holds great promise for real-world clinical applications in disease diagnosis. Its ability to adaptively optimize ensemble weights and size ensures that the diagnostic system is fine-tuned to the specific characteristics of the patient data. This adaptability is crucial in medical settings where patient populations can be diverse and dynamic. By providing accurate and robust diagnostic predictions, the approach can aid clinicians in making more informed decisions, potentially leading to improved patient outcomes.

#### 5.13.1.2 Interpretability and Explainability

Interpretability is a critical aspect of machine learning models applied in clinical settings. As the ensemble consists of multiple base classifiers, understanding the ensemble's decision-making process and the factors contributing to each prediction becomes challenging. Future research should explore techniques to enhance the interpretability and explainability of the Dynamic Weighted Ensemble Approach. Methods such as LIME (Local Interpretable Model-Agnostic Explanations) or SHAP (Shapley Additive exPlanations) can shed light on the factors influencing the ensemble's predictions for individual patients, enabling clinicians to trust and validate the system's outputs.

### 5.13.2 Integration with Decision Support Systems

#### 5.13.2.1 Decision Support Systems in Clinical Practice

Integrating the Dynamic Weighted Ensemble Approach with existing clinical decision support systems can greatly enhance their capabilities. Decision support systems provide valuable insights and recommendations to healthcare professionals, aiding

**TABLE 5.10**
**Comparison between SOTA Ensemble Models and Proposed Model on Various Datasets**

| Dataset | Classifiers | Accuracy | AUC | Sensitivity | Specificity | Reference |
|---|---|---|---|---|---|---|
| | Stacking (LR) | 0.761 | 0.838 | 0.871 | 0.559 | [17] |
| | Adaboost (DS) | 0.750 | 0.810 | 0.849 | 0.566 | [17] |
| | Bagging (4.5) | 0.754 | 0.825 | 0.855 | 0.565 | [17] |
| | Adaboost (C4.5) | 0.725 | 0.780 | 0.804 | 0.578 | [17] |
| | Bagging (L-SVM) | 0.764 | 0.813 | 0.889 | 0.541 | [17] |
| | Bagging (RBF-SVM) | 0.681 | 0.734 | 0.867 | 0.333 | [17] |
| | Majority Voting (MV) | 0.762 | 0.721 | 0.887 | 0.532 | [17] |
| | Bagging (Poly-SVM) | 0.762 | 0.811 | 0.882 | 0.539 | [17] |
| | Stacking (NSGA-II) | 0.838 | 0.859 | 0.961 | 0.791 | [17] |
| PID | Bagging (REP) | 0.758 | 0.832 | 0.837 | 0.611 | [17] |
| | Random Subspace Method (RSM) | 0.753 | 0.827 | 0.869 | 0.542 | [17] |
| | Random Forest | 0.763 | 0.839 | 0.846 | 0.603 | [17] |
| | Stacking | 0.688 | 0.665 | 0.742 | 0.587 | [17] |
| | Dia-Net | 0.908 | - | 0.957 | 0.831 | [1] |
| | Soft-voting | 0.809 | 0.790 | 0.706 | 0.784 | [18] |
| | AdaBoost | 0.749 | 0. | 0.682 | 0.601 | [18] |
| | Bagging | 0.701 | 0.748 | 0.687 | - | [18] |
| | Gradient Boost | 0.718 | 0.753 | 0.487 | - | [18] |
| | XGBoost | 0.691 | 0.757 | 0.675 | - | [18] |
| | CatBoost | 0.745 | 0.753 | 0.650 | - | [18] |
| | **Proposed Approach (10 bags)** | **0.909** | **0.905** | **0.890** | **0.919** | **This study** |
| | **Proposed Approach (5 bags)** | **0.922** | **0.911** | **0.872** | **0.949** | **This study** |
| | Stacking ensemble | 0.923 | 0.922 | 0.934 | 0.910 | [27] |
| | Random Forest | 0.902 | 0.899 | 0.951 | 0.848 | [27] |
| | Extra Tree Classifier | 0.909 | 0.904 | 0.943 | 0.860 | [27] |
| SHD | XGB | 0.919 | 0.917 | 0.943 | 0.892 | [27] |
| | AdaBoost | 0.834 | 0.831 | 0.886 | 0.776 | [27] |
| | GBM | 0.842 | 0.839 | 0.902 | 0.776 | [27] |

**TABLE 5.10 (Continued)**
**Comparison between SOTA Ensemble Models and Proposed Model on Various Datasets**

| Dataset | Classifiers | Accuracy | AUC | Sensitivity | Specificity | Reference |
|---|---|---|---|---|---|---|
| | **Proposed Approach (10 bags)** | **0.907** | **0.889** | **0.809** | **0.969** | **This study** |
| | **Proposed Approach (5 bags)** | **0.907** | **0.906** | **0.904** | **0.909** | **This study** |
| WBC | RF | 0.960 | 0.960 | 0.950 | 0.960 | [19] |
| | Xgboost | 0.970 | 0.970 | 0.950 | 0.990 | [19] |
| | Gradient Boosting | 0.930 | 0.980 | 0.930 | 0.940 | [19] |
| | **Proposed Approach (10 bags)** | **0.991** | **0.988** | **0.976** | **1.00** | **This study** |
| | **Proposed Approach (5 bags)** | **0.982** | **0.981** | **0.976** | **0.985** | **This study** |

in diagnosis, treatment planning, and patient management. By incorporating the ensemble's predictions into such systems, clinicians can benefit from the system's collective intelligence and diverse perspectives, leading to more accurate and reliable decision-making.

#### 5.13.2.2 Real-time and On-demand Diagnostics

Another avenue for future exploration is the development of real-time and on-demand diagnostic systems using the Dynamic Weighted Ensemble Approach. Such systems can be deployed in point-of-care settings, allowing for immediate and continuous diagnostic support. Patients can receive personalized diagnostic predictions based on their data, enabling timely interventions and personalized treatment plans.

### 5.13.3 Further Enhancements and Extensions

#### 5.13.3.1 Robustness and Generalization

Ensuring the robustness and generalization of the Dynamic Weighted Ensemble Approach is essential for its successful deployment in diverse clinical settings. Further research can focus on enhancing the ensemble's ability to handle data from different sources, dealing with missing or noisy data, and addressing concept drift in longitudinal medical data.

**TABLE 5.11**
**Comparison between SOTA Nonensemble Models and Proposed Model on Various Datasets**

| Dataset | Classifier | Accuracy | AUC | Sensitivity | Precision | F1 Score | Ref. |
|---|---|---|---|---|---|---|---|
| PID | SM rule miner | 0.898 | - | **0.946** | - | - | [20] |
| | RST-BAT miner | 0.853 | - | 0.926 | - | - | [21] |
| | LR | 0.751 | - | 0.710 | 0.689 | 0.699 | [22] |
| | DT | 0.668 | - | 0.711 | 0.630 | 0.751 | [22] |
| | MLP | 0.772 | - | 0.525 | 0.682 | 0.590 | [14] |
| | NB | 0.776 | - | 0.661 | 0.759 | 0.707 | [23] |
| | SVM | 0.741 | 0.740 | 0.712 | 0.754 | 0.732 | [23] |
| | KNN | 0.719 | 0.663 | 0.612 | 0.583 | 0.597 | [18] |
| | DT | 0.859 | 0.851 | - | 0.821 | 0.903 | [24] |
| | DCN | 0.862 | 0.912 | 0.842 | 0.819 | - | [25] |
| | C4.5 | 0.751 | 0.792 | 0.829 | 0.716 | 0.768 | [23] |
| | **Proposed Approach (10 bags)** | **0.909** | **0.905** | **0.890** | **0.859** | **0.875** | **This study** |
| | **Proposed Approach (5 bags)** | **0.922** | **0.911** | **0.872** | **0.905** | **0.888** | **This study** |
| SHD | LR | 0.840 | 0.901 | 0.835 | 0.850 | 0.838 | [26] |
| | LDA | 0.840 | 0.906 | 0.835 | 0.850 | 0.838 | [26] |
| | SVM | 0.837 | 0.903 | 0.830 | 0.849 | 0.834 | [26] |
| | MLP | 0.842 | 0.840 | 0.894 | 0.820 | 0.856 | [26] |
| | KNN | 0.808 | 0.805 | 0.869 | 0.786 | 0.826 | [27] |
| | CART | 0.842 | 0.841 | 0.869 | 0.835 | 0.852 | [27] |
| | DBN+CSA | 0.912 | 0.870 | - | - | - | [27] |
| | **Proposed Approach (10 bags)** | **0.907** | **0.889** | **0.809** | **0.944** | **0.871** | **This study** |
| | **Proposed Approach (5 bags)** | **0.907** | **0.906** | **0.904** | **0.863** | **0.883** | **This study** |
| WBC | LR | 0.956 | - | 0.958 | 0.971 | 0.965 | [28] |
| | SVM | 0.971 | - | 0.958 | 0.971 | 0.965 | [28] |
| | KNN | 0.929 | - | 0.916 | 0.970 | 0.942 | [28] |
| | DT | 0.910 | - | 0.910 | 0.910 | 0.910 | [28] |
| | DT | 0.910 | 0.890 | 0.880 | 0.910 | 0.910 | [19] |
| | GNB | 0.940 | 0.940 | 0.930 | 0.940 | 0.940 | [19] |
| | SVM Linear | 0.970 | 0.970 | 0.980 | 0.970 | 0.970 | [19] |
| | SVM RBF | 0.970 | 0.960 | 0.930 | 0.960 | 0.960 | [19] |
| | **Proposed Approach (10 bags)** | **0.991** | **0.988** | **0.976** | **1.00** | **0.988** | **This study** |
| | **Proposed Approach (5 bags)** | **0.982** | **0.981** | **0.976** | **0.976** | **0.976** | **This study** |

#### 5.13.3.2 Semi-supervised and Transfer Learning

Exploring semi-supervised and transfer learning techniques within the context of the Dynamic Weighted Ensemble Approach can be valuable. In medical scenarios, labeled data can be scarce, while unlabeled data may be abundant. Semi-supervised learning can leverage both labeled and unlabeled data to improve model performance. Additionally, transfer learning can facilitate the transfer of knowledge across related disease domains, allowing the ensemble to adapt quickly to new diagnostic tasks.

#### 5.13.3.3 Multi-class and Multi-label Classification

Expanding the Dynamic Weighted Ensemble Approach to handle multi-class and multi-label classification problems is crucial for its broader applicability. Many medical diagnoses involve multiple classes or may require assigning multiple labels to each patient. Extending the approach to accommodate such scenarios would make it more versatile and applicable to a wide range of medical conditions.

## 5.14 CONCLUSION

The proposed Dynamic Weighted Ensemble Approach presents a promising direction for disease diagnosis using ensemble learning and the TLBO algorithm. In this study TLBO optimized the worst bag fitness in every iteration and improved the disease diagnosis predictive performance as well showing improved adaptability, accuracy, and diversity. This makes it a strong candidate for integration into clinical decision support systems, where it can aid clinicians in making more informed and effective decisions. The robustness of the model was evaluated with three benchmark disease datasets: PID, SHD, and WBC. We also evaluated the diversity using different numbers of bags as well as dynamic bag sizes. The results provide strong evidence that the proposed model is effective not only in terms of accuracy and diversity but also across other performance measures such as sensitivity, specificity, and precision. Future research and development efforts should focus on enhancing its interoperability, generalization, and applicability across various clinical settings and diagnostic tasks.

## REFERENCES

1. Ramalingaswamy Cheruku, Damodar Reddy Edla, and Venkatanareshbabu Kuppili. *Soft Computing Techniques for Type-2 Diabetes Data Classification*. CRC Press, 2020.
2. Ramalingaswamy Cheruku and Damodar ReddyEdla. Selector: PSO as model selector for dual-stage diabetes network. *Journal of Intelligent Systems*, 29(1):475–484, 2018.
3. Satyanarayana Nimmala, Y Ramadevi, R Sahith, and Ramalingaswamy Cheruku. High blood pressure prediction based on AAA++ using machine-learning algorithms. *Cogent Engineering*, 5(1):1497114, 2018.
4. Ahsan Hussain, Bettahally N Keshavamurthy, and Ramalingaswamy Cheruku. Dynamic multi-layer ensemble classification framework for social venues using binary particle swarm optimization. *Wireless Personal Communications*, 105(4):1491–1511, 2019.

5. Srinivas Arukonda and Ramalingaswamy Cheruku. A novel stacking framework with pso optimized svm for effective disease classification. *Journal of Intelligent & Fuzzy Systems*, 45(3):4105–4123, 2023.
6. R Venkata Rao, Vimal J Savsani, and DP Vakharia. Teaching–learning-based optimization: A novel method for constrained mechanical design optimization problems. *Computer-aided Design*, 43(3):303–315, 2011.
7. Xibin Dong, Zhiwen Yu, Wenming Cao, Yifan Shi, and Qianli Ma. A survey on ensemble learning. *Frontiers of Computer Science*, 14:241–258, 2020.
8. Krishna Swaroop, Ramalingaswamy Cheruku, and Damoder Reddy Edla. Cascading of RBFN, PNN and SVM for improved type-2 diabetes prediction accuracy. *Australian Journal of Wireless Technologies, Mobility and Security*, 1: 24–27,2019 .
9. Srinivas Arukonda and S Sountharrajan. Investigation of lung cancer detection using 3d convolutional deep neural network. In *2020 2nd International Conference on Advances in Computing, Communication Control and Networking (ICACCCN)*, 763–768. IEEE, 2020.
10. Damodar Edla Ramalingaswamy Cheruku and VenkatanareshbabuKuppili. An optimized and efficient radial basis neural network using cluster validity index for diabetes classification. *Group (cluster),* 7:10, 2019.
11. Shasha Mao, Jia-Wei Chen, Licheng Jiao, Shuiping Gou, and Rongfang Wang. Maximizing diversity by transformed ensemble learning. *Applied Soft Computing*, 82:105580, 2019.
12. Leo Breiman. Bagging predictors. *Machine Learning*, 24(2):123–140, 1996.
13. Robert E Schapire et al. A brief introduction to boosting. *IJCAI*, 99:1401–1406, 1999, Citeseer.
14. Satish Kumar Kalagotla, Suryakanth VGangashetty, and Kanuri Giridhar. A novel stacking technique for prediction of diabetes. *Computers in Biology and Medicine*, 135:104554, 2021.
15. Srinivas Arukonda and Ramalingaswamy Cheruku. A novel diversity-based ensemble approach with genetic algorithm for effective disease diagnosis. *Soft Computing*, 27(14):1–20,2023.
16. Yoonsuh Jung. Multiple predicting k-fold cross-validation for model selection. *Journal of Nonparametric Statistics*, 30(1):197–215, 2018.
17. Namrata Singh and Pradeep Singh. Stacking-based multi-objective evolutionary ensemble framework for prediction of diabetes mellitus. *Biocybernetics and Biomedical Engineering*, 40(1):1–22, 2020.
18. Saloni Kumari, Deepika Kumar, and Mamta Mittal. An ensemble approach for classification and prediction of diabetes mellitus using soft voting classifier. *International Journal of Cognitive Computing in Engineering*, 2:40–46, 2021.
19. Nosayba Al-Azzam and Ibrahem Shatnawi. Comparing supervised and semi-supervised machine learning models on diagnosing breast cancer. *Annals of Medicine and Surgery*, 62:53–64, 2021.
20. Ramalingaswamy Cheruku, Damodar Reddy Edla, and Venkatanareshbabu Kuppili. Sm-ruleminer: Spider monkey based rule miner using novel fitness function for diabetes classification. *Computers in Biology and Medicine*, 81:79–92, 2017.
21. Ramalingaswamy Cheruku, Damodar Reddy Edla, Venkatanareshbabu Kuppili, and Ramesh Dharavath. Rst-batminer: A fuzzy rule miner integrating rough set feature selection and bat optimization for detection of diabetes disease. *Applied Soft Computing*, 67:764–780, 2018.

22. Ibomoiye Domor Mienye and Yanxia Sun. Performance analysis of cost-sensitive learning methods with application to imbalanced medical data. *Informatics in Medicine Un-locked*, 25:100690, 2021.
23. Nur Ulfa Maulidevi, Kridanto Surendro, et al. SMOTE-LOF for noise identification in imbalanced data classification. *Journal of King Saud University-Computer and Information Sciences*, 34(6):3413–3423, 2022.
24. Chandrashekhar Azad, Bharat Bhushan, Rohit Sharma, Achyut Shankar, Krishna Kant Singh, and Aditya Khamparia. Prediction model using smote, genetic algorithm and decision tree (PMSGD) for classification of diabetes mellitus. *Multimedia Systems*, 28(4):1289–1307, 2022.
25. Suja A Alex, J Nayahi, H Shine, and Vaisshalli Gopirekha. Deep convolutional neural network for diabetes mellitus prediction. *Neural Computing and Applications*, 34(2):1319–1327, 2022.
26. Burak Kolukisa and Burcu Bakir-Gungor. Ensemble feature selection and classification methods for machine learning-based coronary artery disease diagnosis. *Computer Standards & Interfaces*, 84:103706,2022.
27. Achyut Tiwari, Aryan Chugh, and Aman Sharma. Ensemble framework for cardiovascular disease prediction. *Computers in Biology and Medicine*, 146:105624,2022.
28. Muhammad Sakib Khan Inan, RizwanHasan, and Fahim IrfanAlam. A hybrid probabilistic ensemble based extreme gradient boosting approach for breast cancer diagnosis. In *2021 IEEE 11th Annual Computing and Communication Workshop and Conference (CCWC)*, 1029–1035. IEEE, 2021.

# 6 Cataloging of Alzheimer's Disease and Its Stages Using Machine Learning

*S. Rajalakshmi, L. Malliga, P. Mathiyalagan, P. Prema, Ms. S. Biruntha, and Rama Abirami K.*

## 6.1 INTRODUCTION

The neurodegenerative state also known as Alzheimer's disease (AD) affects a huge number of people globally. Patients with AD need to be diagnosed and treated as soon as possible to improve their quality of life. A non-invasive imaging method known as magnetic resonance imaging (MRI) can be used to look for the changes in the structure of the brain that relates to AD. In recent years machine learning algorithms have been developed to predict the presence of AD from MRI data. The most common developments in MRI-based machine learning methods for AD diagnosis are discussed in this research. First, there is analysis of studies on the neuroimaging biomarkers that are used to diagnose AD, and then the various machine learning algorithms that are used to diagnose AD are discussed. Finally, the chapter looks at the possible future directions of the various models in research in this field, including the application of personalized medicine and multimodal imaging.

## 6.2 ALZHEIMER'S DISEASE DETECTION TECHNIQUES

Recent advances in technology have enabled the collection of vast amounts of data. AI techniques have been developed to assist in analyzing such data for clinical decision-making and diagnosis. Alzheimer's infection (AD) is the most widely recognized neurodegenerative disorder among older adults. There is a substantial gap between initial onset of AD pathology and clinical diagnosis of AD dementia, which can be definitively confirmed only through post-mortem examination. Thus, it is unquestionably difficult to diagnose early AD with accuracy. So, there is a specific need for methods to aid clinicians in the recognition of this illness. Both inherited and environmental factors, which influence a person's cognition over time, contribute to the development of Alzheimer's disease. A person will develop this sickness because of inherited alterations.


DOI: 10.1201/9781003449058-6

## 6.3 MACHINE LEARNING METHODOLOGY USING CNN WITH RESNET 50 ALGORITHM

### 6.3.1 Challenges of Mild Cognitive Impairment (MCI)

Alzheimer's disease can develop in individuals with Mild Cognitive Impairment (MCI). In many cases, severe MCI leads to dementia as memory loss becomes more significant. During the advanced stages of the disease, complications such as dehydration, malnutrition, or infections may arise, which can ultimately contribute to death [1]. Early identification of MCI helps individuals adopt healthier lifestyle strategies and positive coping approaches to slow the progression of cognitive decline

### 6.3.2 Machine Learning for AD Detection

A potentially effective treatment for AD is early diagnosis and treatment. The diagnosis of AD is challenging, especially in the initial stages. A neuropsychological evaluation is typically used for the early diagnosis of AD [2]. The clinician's skills and expertise will determine how accurate the mental exams are. It will cost more money and take longer to administer this test to a huge number of AD patients. Therefore, it is essential to develop an automated detection and classification strategy. Clinicians are responsible for interpreting medical information, but this task is often difficult because medical images are highly complex and vary widely across individuals. Due to this variability and the demanding nature of image analysis, relying solely on human interpretation can be challenging in real clinical settings. Consequently, the use of AI has emerged as a valuable approach, providing accurate and reliable outputs for clinical data. The rapid advancement of AI algorithms enables the extraction and characterization of high-level features, assisting in the fast and precise diagnosis of Alzheimer's disease (AD). Although no cure for AD currently exists, significant research efforts are focused on developing new clinical interventions that may slow or halt the disease. Since treatment is most effective in the early stages, these interventions target the initial phase of the condition before substantial cellular damage occurs. Because no single amyloid protein has been demonstrated to reliably diagnose the disease, the use of AI (ML) techniques to find appropriate combinations of amyloid proteins in order to recognize AD is a viable methodology.

### 6.3.3 EEG for AD Detection

This approach uses datasets related to early EEG images and Alzheimer's disease. A dataset expansion technique based on a weighted combination of both positive and negative samples has been proposed to achieve more stable and reliable information, along with a classification framework formulated using linear regression. This model helps extract more meaningful image feature representations while strengthening its generalization capability [3]. The conclusion of the Alzheimer's disease model achieves the practical application's influence. Imaging techniques are remarkably helpful in determining the precise endpoint of AD and also in identifying its early preclinical phases. In order to distinguish AD from other illnesses associated with the cerebrum, EEG is the brain imaging technique that is used most frequently. Many techniques are used extensively, including MRI, PET, X-beam computed tomography (CT), single-photon emission computerized tomography (SPECT), and diffusion tensor imaging (DTI). With the advancement of brain imaging technologies, there is increasing interest in component-based techniques such as magnetic resonance imaging (MRI) and fluorodeoxyglucose positron emission tomography (FDG-PET) for assessing the rate of disease progression [4].

### 6.3.4 Middle Stage Prodrome

Typically, the later stage of Alzheimer's disease is considered the most advanced stage, which can last for a very long time. A higher level of care will be necessary when the disease worsens for the Alzheimer's patient. People with Alzheimer's may have trouble speaking, and they may act strangely, such as refusing to wash dishes or becoming confused or irate. Posing opinions and doing errands can be difficult when there is damage to the brain's nerve cells. People often tend to lose the capability to respond to their current situations, to carry out a conversation. Finally, the disease progresses into the final stage of the illness [5]. Even when they attempt to speak, it becomes difficult to express discomfort or pain since they may struggle to use words or meaningful expressions. Critical character changes could occur when memory and mental capacities decline, and broad assistance with everyday exercises might be required. Many individuals with Alzheimer's disease experience behavioral changes such as anxiety, restlessness, aggression, and sleep disturbances, which are often the most challenging and distressing symptoms to manage. These changes can significantly affect the individual's quality of life. Several factors may contribute to such behavioral symptoms. Medication-related causes include side effects of prescription drugs or interactions resulting from taking multiple medications over long periods. Medical conditions, such as infections, can also influence behavior. For example, pneumonia or urinary tract infections may cause discomfort, while untreated ear or sinus infections can lead to dizziness and pain. Environmental factors may further trigger behavioral changes, including relocation to a new home or care facility, misinterpreted threats, or feelings of fear and confusion when trying to navigate a complex environment [6]. Treatments for behavioral symptoms generally fall into two categories: non-drug interventions and prescription medications.

### 6.3.5 Classification of Alzheimer's Disease Using Machine Learning Algorithm

Personalized treatment planning and monitoring are critical components of cancer disease management. Tailoring treatment plans to individual patients can lead to improved outcomes and patient satisfaction. However, achieving this level of personalization requires comprehensive and accurate assessment of disease severities, identification of adverse effects, and consideration of comorbidity conditions.

By understanding the challenges and addressing them effectively, physicians can enhance their ability to provide personalized treatment plans that consider the specific needs and characteristics of each patient. Accurate prognosis tracking and adverse effect monitoring contribute to treatment optimization, allowing healthcare professionals to make well-informed decisions that maximize efficacy while minimizing potential risks.

### 6.3.6 IoT-Relevant Healthcare Data and Data Integration Challenges

The rise of the Internet of Things (IoT) has brought about significant advancements in healthcare, generating vast amounts of data from various sources such as wearable devices, remote monitoring systems, and sensor-equipped medical devices. This IoT-relevant healthcare data holds immense potential for improving patient care, enabling early detection of diseases, and facilitating real-time monitoring of health conditions. However, integrating this diverse and voluminous data into existing healthcare systems poses considerable challenges.

One major challenge is data interoperability, as IoT devices and systems often employ different communication protocols and data formats. The lack of standardization and compatibility hampers the seamless integration of IoT-generated data into the healthcare ecosystem. Healthcare professionals must grapple with the task of harmonizing and integrating data from different IoT devices to obtain a comprehensive view of the patient's health status.

In particular, image data plays a vital role in diagnosing and monitoring various diseases. However, integrating image data into healthcare systems presents additional challenges. Medical images are typically large, complex, and require specialized software for analysis. Furthermore, the integration of image data with other patient information, such as electronic health records and laboratory results, can be arduous due to the need for efficient storage, transmission, and retrieval of these data types.

Addressing these challenges requires innovative approaches to data integration. Standardization efforts, such as the use of common data models and interoperability standards, can facilitate the seamless exchange and integration of IoT-relevant healthcare data. Additionally, advanced technologies such as artificial intelligence and machine learning can aid in automating the integration process, extracting meaningful insights from diverse datasets, and supporting clinical decision-making.

By overcoming the challenges related to data interoperability and image data integration, healthcare professionals can unlock the full potential of IoT-relevant data in improving patient care, early disease detection, and personalized treatment strategies.

### 6.3.7 Overview of the Need for Integrated Tools that Leverage Ontologies

To overcome the challenges faced by physicians in prognosis tracking, adverse effect monitoring, and personalized treatment planning, the integration of tools that leverage ontologies is crucial. Ontologies provide a structured representation of medical knowledge, standardized terminologies, and semantic relationships. Integrating ontologies with data sources allows for a more intuitive and efficient retrieval and analysis process.

Semantic technologies, such as ontologies, enable the integration of disparate data sources by harmonizing and standardizing terminology. They facilitate the linking of diagnostic summaries, disease severities, adverse effects, and comorbidity conditions with patient-specific characteristics, treatments, and outcomes. By leveraging semantic technologies, physicians gain access to a unified and holistic view of patient data, enabling more efficient decision-making, personalized treatment planning, and monitoring of adverse effects.

However, by leveraging semantic technologies and integrating tools that utilize ontologies, physicians can overcome these challenges. The use of ontologies facilitates the integration and standardization of diverse data sources, improving data retrieval and analysis. The next section explores how semantic technologies can be helpful in addressing these challenges and enhancing cancer disease management practices.

## 6.4 CLASSIFICATION OF ALZHEIMER'S DISEASE USING MACHINE LEARNING ALGORITHM

The suggested method makes use of CNN with RESNET 50 computation. In addition to helping to accurately identify this infection, the employment of AI techniques in conjunction with radiographic (EEG) scanning can also be reliable in resolving the problem of a shortage of qualified medical practitioners in remote networks. The Adam enhancer is combined with an absolute cross-entropy model. The task of predicting a dependent variable's value (y) in light of a specific autonomous variable is carried out by straight relapse (x). Thus, this relapse method identifies a clear relationship between x (information) and y (yield). The best-performing trained model is then used as both the training and testing reference for the prediction framework, employing the proposed CNN with the ResNet-50 architecture.

The chaotic neural network is then used to evaluate and predict whether the input belongs to a dementia patient or a non-dementia individual. The performance of the model is assessed using metrics such as precision, recall, and F1-score across multiple thresholds. To identify if the precision and the result achieved is higher than the pre-existing computation, we use the Python recovery and reconstruction approach. The present framework includes SVM [7]. Our improvements in precision and use of the linear relapse calculation are the results of our advancements. Alzheimer's disease (AD) is a neurodegenerative disorder characterized by cognitive impairments, difficulties in performing daily activities, and socially disruptive behaviors. Electroencephalogram (EEG) signals have been widely used to study and diagnose dementia in clinical and research settings [8].

### 6.4.1 Modules

#### 6.4.1.1 Training Model

The training samples are augmented using transformations such as horizontal flipping, width shifting, and height shifting. During rotation-based augmentation, some pixels may move outside the original image boundary, creating empty regions that must be filled using appropriate interpolation techniques.

#### 6.4.1.2 Pre-Processing

Pre-processing of information, which is a crucial step in the data mining process, refers to the control or removal of information prior to its use to ensure or improve performance. Big data analysis and AI initiatives are good examples of when the phrase "garbage in, garbage out" is applicable. here because Information gathering techniques are often over controlled, resulting in out-of-range values, confusing information blends, missing attributes, etc., the crude information for primary EEG reports. For our examination, we have done some pre-processing of the information [9]. The pre-processing steps of the dataset occur before handing it to the proposed system [10].

#### 6.4.1.3 Feature Extraction

The normal subspace will be smaller as a result of the element vectors for typical Alzheimer's having largely consistent properties. The subspace representing the shared knowledge is learned using these feature vectors. Feature extraction, a key step in the dimensionality reduction process, involves partitioning and condensing high-dimensional data into more compact and meaningful representations. Figure 6.1 will show the proposed architecture, cataloging AD and its stages.

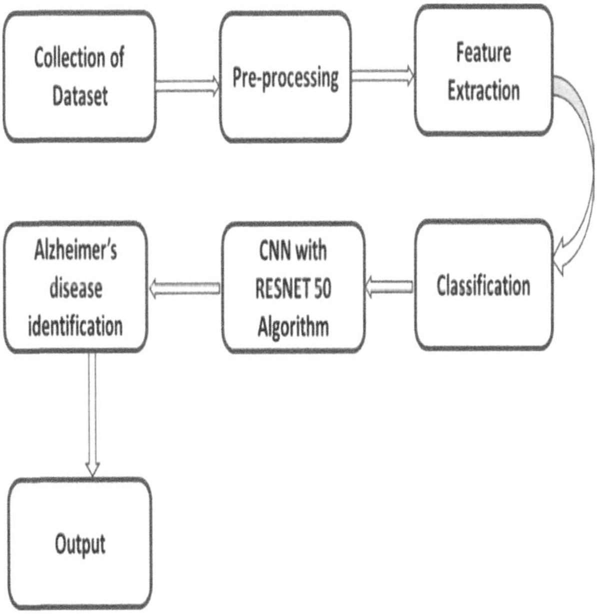


**FIGURE 6.1** Proposed architecture.

#### 6.4.1.4 Epoch Value Generation

In a processing environment, age is typically computed through a comparison of time and date values, although the system clock and timestamps of a computer may not always be perfectly accurate. Age is often referenced relative to Coordinated Universal Time (UTC) at a specific date and at 00:00:00, although this reference point may vary across different systems. By considering these temporal attributes and their coordination, the age value can be accurately derived, enabling both training and testing datasets to be generated.

#### 6.4.1.5 Classification

For each data point in the dataset, the classification method predicts the corresponding target class. By analyzing patterns of disease, the classification strategy can be used to associate a risk factor with individual patients. The model delivers an accuracy of 85% in determining whether a condition is present or not. Table 6.1 shows the comparison of CNN-RESNET 50 with KNN, DT, and RF for accuracy and epoch value.

### 6.4.2 Proposed Algorithm

CNN with RESNET 50, a Convolutional Neural Network (CNN) with the ResNet50 algorithm can be used to classify Alzheimer's disease and its stages using machine learning.

ResNet50 is a pre-trained CNN architecture that consists of 50 convolutional layers, which are designed to extract increasingly complex features from images. This architecture has been trained on a large dataset of images and can be fine-tuned for specific classification tasks.

In the context of Alzheimer's disease classification, the CNN with ResNet50 algorithm processes MRI brain images to detect patterns and features that are indicative of Alzheimer's disease and its stages. The input image is fed into the network, and the network applies a series of convolutions and pooling operations to extract features from the image. The resulting feature map is then fed into a fully connected layer, which produces a probability distribution over the possible classes (e.g., healthy control, mild cognitive impairment, Alzheimer's disease).

**TABLE 6.1**
**Algorithm Comparison**

| ALGORITHM | ACCURACY | EPOCH |
|---|---|---|
| CNN with RESNET 50 | 95 | 91 |
| KNN | 93 | 89 |
| DT | 94 | 87 |
| RF | 91 | 84 |

During the training process, the network learns to recognize patterns in the input data that are associated with Alzheimer's disease and its stages. The network can then be used to classify new MRI brain images as healthy control, mild cognitive impairment, or Alzheimer's disease with a high degree of accuracy.

Overall, CNN with ResNet50 algorithm is a powerful tool for the classification of Alzheimer's disease and its stages using machine learning, and it has the potential to improve diagnosis and treatment of this devastating disease.

### 6.4.3 Mathematical Formulas

#### 6.4.3.1 Forward Pass

During the forward pass, the input data is fed through the network and transformed by a series of matrix multiplications and nonlinear activation functions. The output of each layer is computed as follows:

$$Z = XW + B \tag{6.1}$$

$$A = \text{activation function } (Z)$$

where X is the input data, W is the weight matrix for the layer, B is the bias vector for the layer, Z is the output of the linear transformation, and A is the output of the activation function.

#### 6.4.3.2 Convolution Operation

The convolution operation involves sliding a filter over the input data and computing the dot product between the filter and the input at each position. The output of the convolution operation can be computed as follows:

$$Y[i,j] = \text{sum}(\text{sum}(X[i:i+f, j:j+f] * F)) + b \tag{6.2}$$

where X is the input data, F is the filter, b is the bias term, f is the filter size, and Y is the output feature map.

### 6.4.4 Dataset

The input dataset used in this model consists of 6400EEG scan images which include all four stages, namely Moderate Demented, Mild Demented, Very Mild Demented and Non-Demented. Figure 6.2 shows the sample demented Alzheimer's scan and Non-Demented Alzheimer's scan dataset.

## 6.5 ARCHITECTURE AND ITS IMPLICATION USING RESNET 50

The improved CNN with RESNET 50 framework can accurately and simultaneously segment Alzheimer, as demonstrated by extensive experiments on the

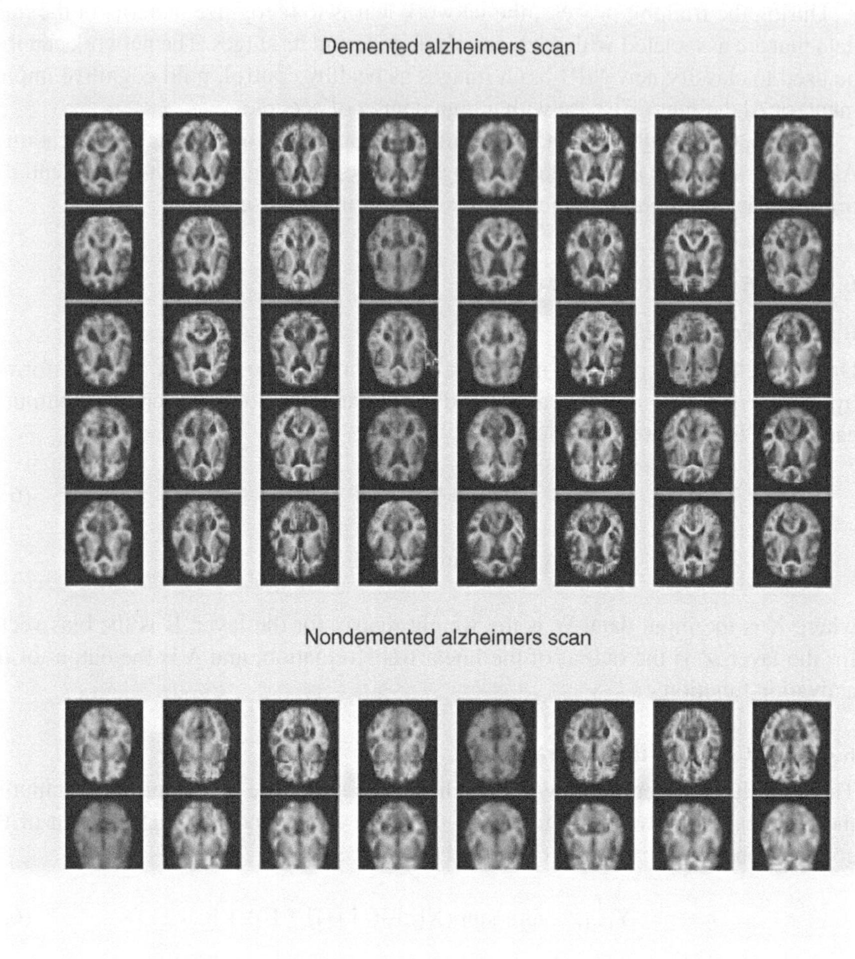


**FIGURE 6.2** Demented Alzheimer's scan and Non-Demented Alzheimer's scan dataset. (The dataset is from Kaggle.)

annotated and collected Alzheimer dataset. In the future, the research can be extended to investigate semi-supervised and weakly supervised methods of brain and organ segmentation because labeling of medical images takes a huge amount of effort and time.

Figure 6.3 shows the accuracy comparison graph. Figure 6.4 shows the confusion matrix in the proposed system provides the result with highest accuracy rate of 97.36%. It classifies the numbers of images in all four stages.

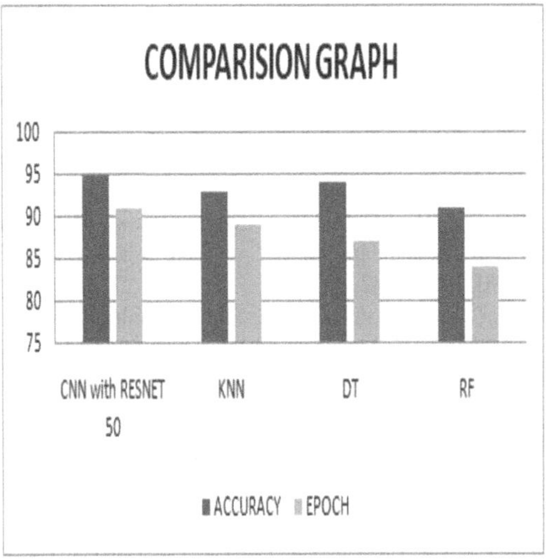


**FIGURE 6.3** Accuracy comparison graph.

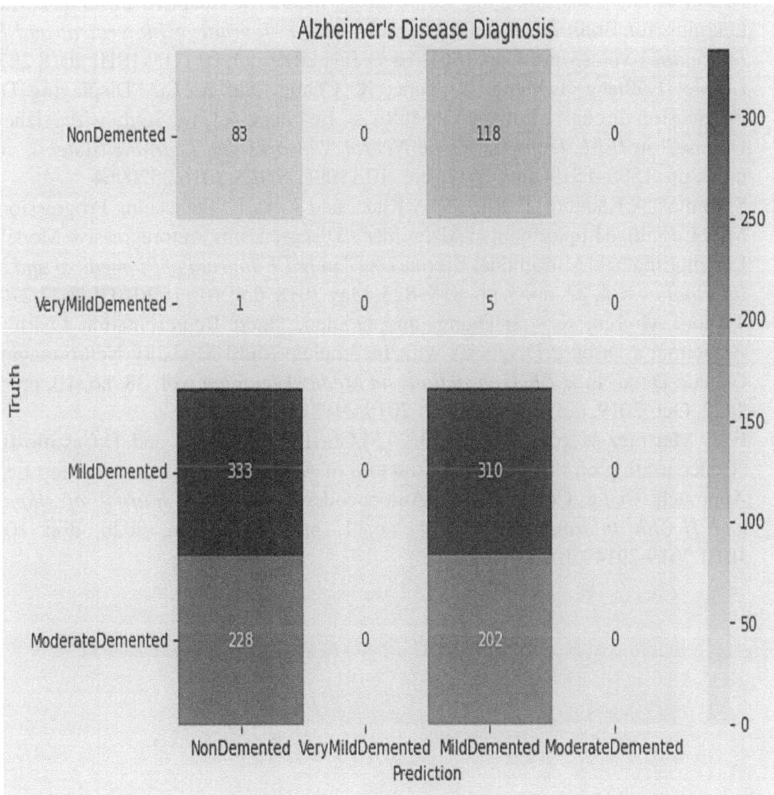


**FIGURE 6.4** Confusion matrix.

## REFERENCES


1. L. Brand, K. Nichols, H. Wang, L.Shen, and H. Huang, "Joint Multi-Modal Longitudinal Regression and Classification for Alzheimer's Disease Prediction," in *IEEE Transactions on Medical Imaging*, vol. 39, no. 6, pp. 1845–1855, June 2020, doi: 10.1109/TMI.2019.2958943
2. R. Cui and M. Liu, "Hippocampus Analysis by Combination of three dimensional DenseNet and Shapes for Alzheimer's Disease Diagnosis," in *IEEE Journal of Biomedical and Health Informatics*, vol. 23, no. 5, pp. 2099–2107, Sept. 2019, doi: 10.1109/JBHI.2018.2882392.
3. M. Dadar et al., "Approval of a Regression Technique for Segmentation of White Matter Hyperintensities in Alzheimer's Disease," in *IEEE Transactions on Medical Imaging*, vol. 36, no. 8, pp. 1758–1768, Aug. 2017, doi: 10.1109/TMI.2017.2693978.
4. B. Jie, M. Liu, J. Liu, D. Zhang, and D. Shen, "Transiently Constrained Group Sparse Learning for Longitudinal Data Analysis in Alzheimer's Disease," in *IEEE Transactions on Biomedical Engineering*, vol. 64, no. 1, pp. 238–249, Jan. 2017, doi: 10.1109/TBME.2016.2553663.
5. P. Jiang, X. Wang, Q. Li, L. Jin, and S. Li, "Connection Aware Sparse and Low-Rank Constrained Multi-Task Learning for Longitudinal Analysis of Alzheimer's Disease," in *IEEE Journal of Biomedical and Health Informatics*, vol. 23, no. 4, pp. 1450–1456, July 2019, doi: 10.1109/JBHI.2018.2885331.
6. B. Lei et al., "Neuroimaging Retrieval by means of Adaptive Ensemble Manifold Learning for Brain Disease Diagnosis," in *IEEE Journal of Biomedical and Health Informatics*, vol. 23, no. 4, pp. 1661–1673, July 2019, doi: 10.1109/JBHI.2018.2872581.
7. L. Nie, L.Zhang, L.Meng, X. Tune, X. Chang, and X. Li, "Displaying Disease Progression through Multisource Multitask Learners: A Case Study with Alzheimer's Disease," in *IEEE Transactions on Neural Networks and Learning Systems*, vol. 28, no. 7, pp. 1508–1519, July 2017, doi: 10.1109/TNNLS.2016.2520964.
8. S.Minhas, A.Khanum, F. Riaz, S. A.Khan, and A.Alvi, "Foreseeing Progression from Mild Cognitive Impairment to Alzheimer's Disease Using Autoregressive Modeling of Longitudinal and Multimodal Biomarkers," in *IEEE Journal of Biomedical and Health Informatics*, vol. 22, no. 3, pp. 818–825, May 2018, doi: 10.1109/JBHI.2017.2703918.
9. T.Zhou, M. Liu, K. - H.Thung, and D.Shen, "Inert Representation Learning for Alzheimer's Disease Diagnosis with Incomplete Multi-Modality Neuroimaging and Genetic Data," in *IEEE Transactions on Medical Imaging*, vol. 38, no. 10, pp. 2411–2422, Oct. 2019, doi: 10.1109/TMI.2019.2913158.
10. F. J. Martinez-Murcia, A.Ortiz, J. - M.Gorriz, J.Ramirez, and D.Castillo-Barnes, "Concentrating on the Manifold Structure of Alzheimer's Disease: A Deep Learning Approach Using Convolutional Autoencoders," in *IEEE Journal of Biomedical and Health Informatics*, vol. 24, no. 1, pp. 17–26, Jan. 2020, doi: 10.1109/JBHI.2019.2914970.

# 7 COVID-19 Fake News Detection to Combat and Mitigate Its Spread

*J. Anuradha, Nalini N., and Sadhanaa Balaji*

## 7.1 INTRODUCTION

At the end of 2019, there were reports of an epidemic outbreak caused by a disease of unknown origin that presented symptoms similar to pneumonia. Most of those infected experienced mild to moderate respiratory illness and recovered without requiring special treatment, while severe cases needed urgent medical attention. COVID-19 became the third major pandemic caused by a deadly virus and had a massive impact in more than 209 countries, including India. According to the WHO, the spread of fake news is considered as dangerous as the spread of COVID-19. Fake news is fabricated news that is deliberately constructed to gain the readers' attention for profit in terms of fame, money, likes, and subscriptions [1]. In due time, social media has become an important tool for both the distribution of information and technological developments and smart devices. The spread of content in social media cannot be controlled. Hence, fake news can reach a large number of people without any restrictions and it not possible to determine the source of information. Fake news involves the spread of violent events happening in the world that disrupt community peace. Figure 7.1 represents the relationship between fake news, rumors, and authentic news. Rumors and fake news are unavoidable; they are always a part of news and are challenging to identify and separate from the authentic news. According to Melissa Zimdars of Merrimack College, who teaches courses such as Introduction to media, fake news can be broadly classified into four categories.

- *Type 1*: Misleading websites are spread in social media to 'outrage' with catchy headlines in order to generate likes, more subscribers, and profit.
- *Type 2*: The spread of unreliable and false information.
- *Type 3*: Sources with clickbait.
- *Type 4*: Sites with sarcasm often have critical comments but pretend to be real.

The spread of misinformation during the outbreak of Ebola at Congo created social disturbance and assaults on many healthcare professionals [3]. In 2002–2003, the SARS epidemic caused uncertainty, and the spread of false information regarding the outbreak gave a wrong notion about Asians. A report published by the *American Journal of Tropical Medicine and Hygiene* revealed that nearly 5000 members were

DOI: 10.1201/9781003449058-7

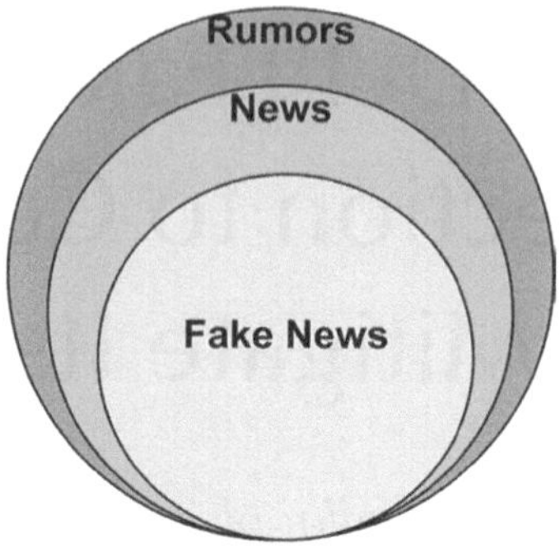


**FIGURE 7.1** Fake news [2].

admitted due to inappropriate and false information on social media [4]. The spread of false information has grown to such an extent that this unreliable information is now being referred to as a new set of misinformation that has accompanied the COVID-19 pandemic: a ‘disinfodemic’ [5]. The disinfodemic has resulted in the sale of herbal products and other fake treatments [6].

Digital platforms are loaded with a lot of feeds on COVID-19. However, few pieces of information shared are true, while a large number of it is fake news and rumors. The spread of fake news and false information has caused an economic drop in a few countries. This has led to some weird behaviors among people in a few countries, such as the non-consumption of animal foods due to an assumption that the virus will spread through animal products. However, critical thinking is seen as an effective weapon to eradicate the spread of fake news [7]. Since the spread of false information affects the security and privacy of the users, there is a demand for developing a robust model that can identify false news. Fake information and assumptions about COVID-19 have been widely spread all over social media and fake cures, such as gargling with lemon or salt water and injecting yourself with bleach, have been promoted as able to kill the virus and other causative microbes [6]. False theories have spread, such as the virus was produced and bioengineered in a lab at Wuhan and is a weapon for bio war [8], or that the 5G cellular networks are causing symptoms similar to that of the coronavirus [9]. An intriguing movie named ‘Plandemic’ was released online in 2020, which immediately drew the attention of a large number of people and gained many views. It became one of the fastest modes of spreading misinformation about the COVID-19 pandemic [10]. A survey conducted by the United Kingdom government found that nearly 46% of the population had been the victims of COVID fake news. Pew research in the United States found similar, here 48% were victims [11]. A YouGov survey had found that 50% of the Fox News viewers and 28% of Americans thought that Bill Gates was planning to use the COVID-19 vaccine to invent and insert microchips in people for the direct detection of the virus in the body [12].

Digital platforms want to achieve the highest numbers of user hits for the monetary benefits. Digital content is made to be sensational, emotional, appeal to sympathy, religious belief, etc., to gain the attention of the users. Social media are the game changers in many domains like politics, film industry, health care, etc. Attacks on medical professional have become quite common due to partial knowledge or misinformation by the digital media. It is often difficult for an individual to verify the validity of the news. It is often more convincing, even from a logical standpoint to believe information that appears factual, even if it is not real. People are susceptible to believing in 'facts' that support their beliefs and then spread them to further users without understanding the underlying purpose.

The spread of fake news is an important problem that needs to be dealt immediately and eradicated as it can harm the public sphere, democracy, freedom of speech and expression, and journalism. Previous literature has shown that New Media Literacy and critical thinking are seen as a survival kit, and are the most essential cognitive tools that individuals can use to protect themselves from fake news on social media. For critical thinkers, all the assumptions are equally questionable and various ideas are welcomed. Such critical thinkers are always willing to inquire, and this inquiry is not affected by their emotions, or prejudices and are not biased in favor of a single outcome. The medium of fake news can be text, video, audio, and images. Some of the various approaches in the spread of fake news are as follows:

- *Visual based*: Misleading information can be in the form of images or videos. Lots of home remedy videos and images were shared for the COVID treatment
- *User based*: The news targets particular types of users based on the age, gender, religion, location, etc.
- *Knowledge based*: Unconventional methods on COVID treatment were stated with few case studies which made the users believe the approach.
- *Style-based journalism*: Adapts the style of accredited journalist to reach the users with misleading facts
- *Sentence based*: It is a form of representing a valid statement. However, its intentions and meaning are different.

Fake news detection can be automated using computational intelligence techniques that include Machine Learning (ML), Deep Learning (DL), Natural Language Processing (NLP), and Social Network Analysis. The dataset curated for such study is a combination of real and fake news that are collected from various digital sources. Preprocessing activity of data cleaning is performed by removing URLs, stop words, and irrelevant data. Data is tokenized and each of these tokens (i.e. features) are evaluated. Features of least importance are discarded for further processing. The refined set of features is trained using ML or DL algorithms to classify the feeds as fake or real.

Fake new detection techniques can be broadly classified into five categories [13].

- Content based
- Context based
- Propagation based

- Multi label learning based
- Hybrid based

## 7.2 LITERATURE REVIEW

The pandemic has fueled the political battle on government health care policies, interpretation of medicine, death claims, and rates of spread. The public are often disturbed by unreliable sources of information with trauma, expression, and grief. The study on the Chinese population revealed that over 70% of the population was affected with psychological distress, with symptoms including anxiety, depression, and insomnia [14]. This has led to a lot of confusion and conflict amongst the people, and conspiracies caused due to the misinformation. A survey of 502 adults by the Centers for Disease Control and Prevention (CDC) in the United States revealed that 39% of people engaged in weird practices like washing food products with bleach, applying household cleaners to skin, and intentionally inhaling or ingesting disinfectants with the goal of preventing viral infection [14].

It was observed that countries with less use of social media were the receivers of the main source of real information and had less trust in social media content. In such countries, it was observed that the mortality rate was lower [15]. Out of Chile, Argentina, Brazil, Colombia and Peru, the countries with the highest exposure to social media were Chile and Argentina, also having the greatest internet reliability rates (92.4% and 92.0%, respectively). They had the highest rates of users browsing COVID-related information in social media networks (32.0% and 28.0%, respectively). Brazil and Colombia had moderate levels of users on social media accessing information about the pandemic. Mexico showed the highest use of social networks, while Peru and Colombia had the highest rate of an inability to recognize fake news and miscommunication [15].

Fake news has received a lot of global attention in the past years. Fake news has entered into all scholarly discourses and in everyday business conversations. AI-based agents like bots were deployed for the creation of fake information during the pandemic outbreak. Deep learning algorithms play an important role in strengthening AI in most of the applications. NLP adds more knowledge to present or interpret the information in native language. This attracts readability by a large population. Powerful deep learning techniques are applied to identify susceptible and false news. These models are deployed for the early detection of the spread of misinformation. The journal *Frontiers in Public Health* has published numerous competitions, dataset, and research articles related to Fake News Detection. Learning Models include transfer learning, bidirectional encoders with transfer learning, ensemble approach, sentiment analysis, RNN, LSTM, and GRU. Bio Medical Information Extraction has considered 1164 news feeds for training the ML model. From which, the 158 best features were selected and applied to 15 different models. Random Forest has achieved the best classification in biomedical data for fake news prediction [16].

A reverse tracking technique was attempted to detect the spread and the origin of misinformation. Ko et al. (2019) applied this technique using a cognitive-based intelligent system for fake news detection.

Manipulation is the disruption or change of beliefs of the real images or videos to create a false condition about the situation [5]. News fabrication is confined to the text-based items, whereas manipulation is defined as the visual news that is presented to the viewer. The study of fake news detection requires lot of evaluations through machine learning techniques on a wide range of datasets [18]. With the advent and invention of modern digital technologies, it allows the conducting of operations over photo and video material, where manipulation has become an easier and more efficient way to spread fake news and miscommunication. A systemic literature search and analysis assists in providing knowledge of the studies and other kinds of literature published on this topic and the false news related to it. This chapter focuses on the following topics.

- Case study of the fake news related to COVID and its impact.
- Fake news detection using NLP and Machine Learning.
- Fake news detection using social network analysis.
- Ways to manage theCOVID-19 infodemic.

## 7.3 FAKE NEWS DATA SET

Text shared in social media related to COVID has been collected from Twitter (now X), Instagram, Facebook, websites, etc. For example, in Twitter the text related to tweets, retweets, user profiles, tweet ids, and news body for every news article is curated to construct the data set. The validity is verified from websites like Boomlive, Poynter, PolitiFact, and Snopes, and it helps to label the news as fake or real. Some of the benchmark datasets used for Fake News detection for COVID-19 are listed in Table1.1.

**TABLE 7.1**
**Fake News Detection Datasets and their Sources**

| Dataset | Source |
|---|---|
| COVID-19 Fake News Dataset | https://paperswithcode.com/dataset/covid-19-fake-news-dataset |
| COVID-19 Fake News Dataset NLP | www.kaggle.com/datasets/elvinagammed/covid19-fake-news-dataset-nlp |
| MM-COVID (Multilingual and Multi dimensional COVID-19 Fake News Data Repository) | https://paperswithcode.com/dataset/mm-covid |
| COVID 19 Dataset | www.ecdc.europa.eu/en/covid-19/data |
| CoAID | https://paperswithcode.com/dataset/coaid |
| CMU-MisCOV19 | https://zenodo.org/record/4024154 |
| FakeCOVID | www.kaggle.com/datasets/arashnic/covid19-fake-news |
| FibVID | https://github.com/merry555/FibVID |

## 7.4 FAKE NEWS DETECTION USING ML AND NLP TECHNIQUES

Spreading false information about COVID-19 on social media platforms has created widespread fear among people. This confusion could result in additional problems. In South Africa, individuals were advised to refuse all COVID-19 tests as it was believed that this action would inadvertently encourage the virus's transmission. Consequently, a number of people expressed objections to undergo COVID-19 examinations. The authorities subsequently released a fake news warning, resulting in the arrest of an individual for creating and disseminating false information (see Figure 7.2). Hence, the detection of fake news is very important. This section discusses the use of machine learning and deep learning methods for detecting fake news.

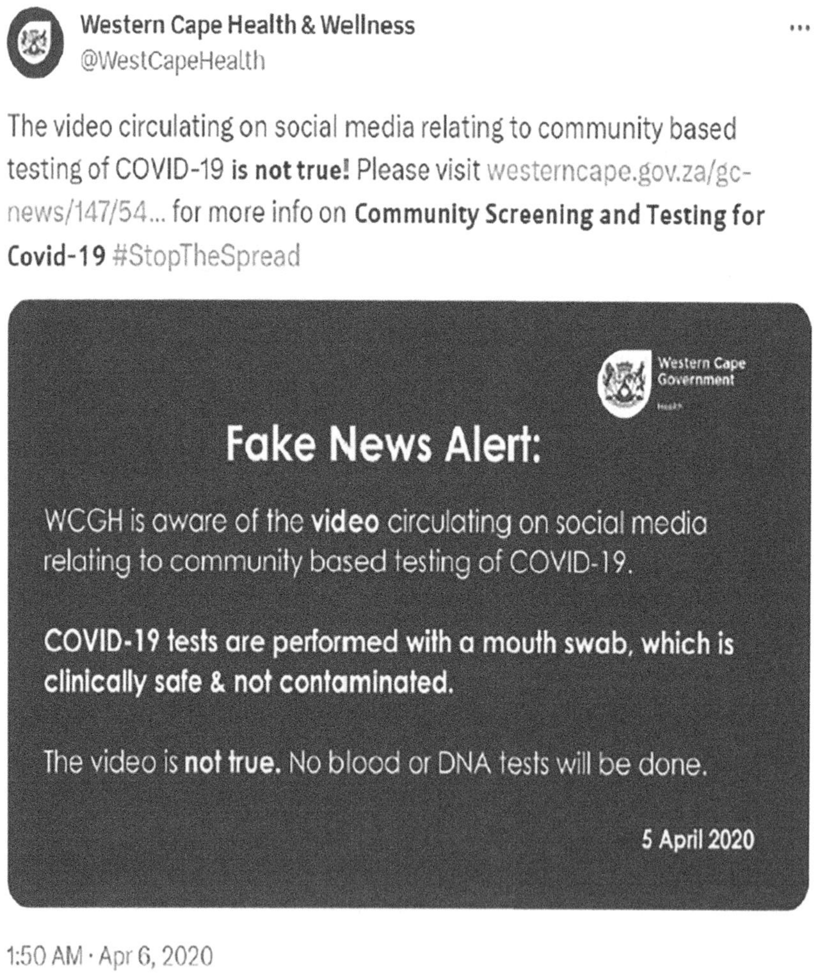


**FIGURE 7.2** Fake news alert by South African Government [17].

The major issues nowadays are the purposeful or unintentional spread of false information. The user finds it difficult to distinguish between authentic and fraudulent news, hence the creation of an intelligent system is necessary. There are many strategies that have been created that offer cutting-edge ways to find harmful information. It is regarded as a classification issue where labels are intended to be connected to specific claims or posts and indicate whether they are accurate or incorrect. As mentioned by the preceding study, the classification methods are further separated into approaches based on machine learning (ML) and deep learning (DL).

### 7.4.1 Machine Learning Techniques to Handle Fake News

Machine Learning techniques are successful in solving many real-world problems. Many of the Machine Learning-based Natural Language Processing (NLP) techniques have been proposed to detect false information in social media and news articles. These algorithms were used to check trustworthiness on COVID-19 related news articles and social media posts. Figure 7.3 depicts the general workflow of ML-based NLP algorithms. The steps involved in this workflow are as follows:

- The dataset was collected from various websites and social media platforms.
- As part of data preprocessing, empty columns, punctuation, and URLs are eliminated from the dataset.
- Tokenization is a procedure used to divide lengthy texts into words or short lines following text preparation.
- Identify the most significant attributes within the dataset.
- Then, the most advanced ML learning methods were used to train the model with features that were extracted.
- Machine Learning models are assessed for their performance using standard metrics.

Castillo et al. [19] proposed a Support Vector Machine (SVM)-based ML model for fake news detection. The method evaluates the credibility of tweets using content- and context-based features. The Graph kernel-based SVM approach is implemented

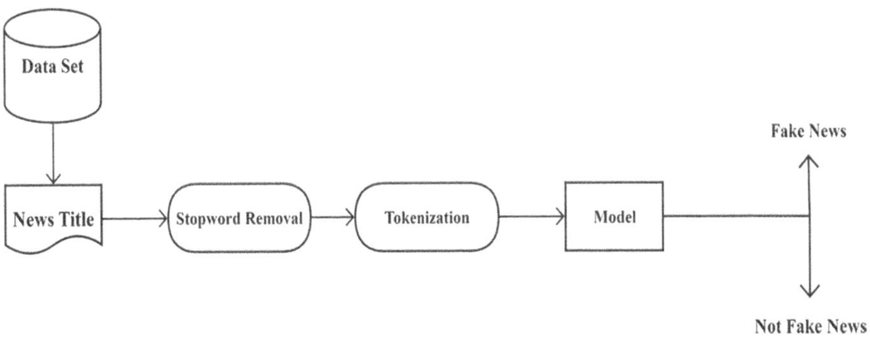


**FIGURE 7.3** General workflow of machine learning algorithms to identify false news.

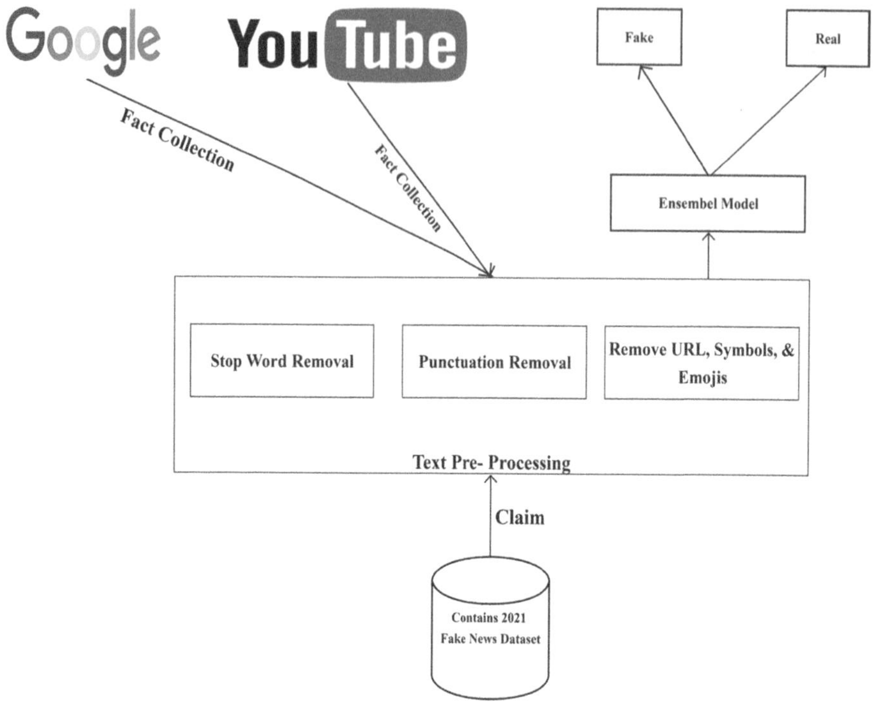


**FIGURE 7.4** Ensemble based model to predict fake news on COVID 19 data.

to identify rumors by analyzing propagation structure and content-based attributes within the Sina-Weibo dataset [20]. Like SVM, logistic regression, Random Forest, and decision tree techniques were used to detect fake news.

Varshney and Vishwakarma (2023) proposed an ensemble model for predicting misleading information during theCOVID-19 pandemic period [21]. They designed a novel voting architecture for several web platforms comprising four distinct sets of innovative attributes: sentiments, content, linguistics, and similarity. These attributes were aggregated from various web platforms to authenticate the news. By employing particular queries and attributes extracted from each hint or headline, an exclusive source platform was formulated to extract pertinent clues or headlines from two web platforms, namely YouTube and Google. The Automatic Multi Web Platform Voting Framework introduced by Varshney and Vishwakarma aims to forecast the dissemination of deceptive information during the COVID-19 pandemic. Figure 7.4 shows the ensemble-based framework of the proposed model. This framework works in two phases.

The first phase performs data gathering, query formulation, fact compilation, and information filtration on the CONSTRAINT 2021 dataset (see Table 7.2). This dataset contains 5000 real samples and 5000 fake samples. In this phase, the data set is pre-processed and cleaned. Subsequently, a query is created by appending the term "fake news," with a space in between. This query is then employed within a Multi

**TABLE 7.2**
**Sample Labels of CONSTRAINT 2021 Dataset**

| Label | Text |
|---|---|
| Fake | Chlorine dioxide generated sodium chloride natural zeolite can cure corona or any virus |
| Real | Breathlessness excessive fatigue and muscle aches from COVID can last for months. |
| Fake | Have ginger boiled in water for 30 min and haldi powder with milk no corona-can touch you. |
| Fake | Try using UV light it kills corona virus and keep you safe |
| Real | Wash your hands often with soap and water for at least 20 sec especially after being in a public place or after blowing your nose coughing or sneezing |
| Real | Avoid touching your eyes nose and mouth with unwashed hands. |
| Real | Coronavirus is a respiratory virus which spreads primarily through droplets generated when an infected person coughs or sneezes or through droplets of saliva or discharge from the nose |

Web platform to fetch pertinent data associated with the constructed query. Using the Selenium Python package, the top ten title headings are then extracted automatically from both platforms. Finally, the algorithm checks the facts and conspiracy in the COVID-related news articles.

In the second phrase, the process involves extraction and classification of clues. This module uses the information gathered in the first phase to extract some useful clues that may be used to determine whether a claim is true or false. The features are classified into four categories: content, linguistic/semantic signals, similarity, and sentiments. The features based on linguistics encompass attributes derived from NLTK POS tagging and semantic similarity, while the content-based features consider factors such as the count of question marks and fabricated words. The cosine similarity is used to calculate how similar two sentences are to one another. Sentiment-based features provide a good, negative, or neutral response to the user's query. These are all indicators of susceptibility to COVID-19 disinformation. To categorize news as misleading or accurate, an ensemble approach using machine learning models is applied. Voting is used to authenticate the news and evaluate the trust or support exhibited by different websites.

The evaluation of the model primarily focused on four metrics: Precision, Recall, F1-score, and Accuracy. These metrics have been used to verify the performance of ensemble-based classification methods, such as Random Forest, SVM and logistic regression. The ensemble-based voting classifiers have demonstrated notably good performance compared to other classifiers and achieved an F1-score of 0.989.

### 7.4.2 Deep Learning Techniques to Handle Fake News

Deep learning (DL) is a subset of machine learning designed to mimic the learning process of the human brain. A notable advantage of DL compared to traditional ML methods is its efficiency in feature extraction, as it reduces the reliance on manually crafted features, resulting in shorter processing times. Moreover, the deep learning framework can be employed to acquire intricate representations from more straightforward inputs that exhibit variations in both context and content. Among the prominent techniques within DL are Convolutional Neural Networks (CNN), Recurrent Neural Networks (RNN), Long Short-Term Memory (LSTM), and Bidirectional Encoder Representations from Transformers (BERT).

Devlin et al. proposed an NLP model on BERT which can be used to identify COVID-19-related misinformation [22]. A pre-trained BERT model was developed using a huge text corpus with an unsupervised approach with deep learning. Since BERT requires a lot of processing, it may be challenging to implement it without specialized computational resources.

Deepak and Chitturi [23] introduced a hybrid model that merged a Feed-forward Neural Network (FNN) with LSTM [23]. This method considers news domains, news writers, and headlines to evaluate the effectiveness of false news identification. They employed word embeddings like Bag of Words (BoW), Word2Vec, and GloVe in combination with LSTM and FNN. The model's results still did not exhibit significant superiority.

Ayoub Jackie et al. [24] developed a distilBERT model which is integrated with SHAP (SHapley Additive exPlanations) to enhance the model's credibility. The attributes are evaluated to get their contribution through SHAP, employing the Shapley value derived from cooperative game theory. Local precision, missing values, and consistency are a few of the important desirable features that make it a good choice for refining machine learning models. Figure 7.5 shows a summary of the distilBERT using SHAP model. This model employs the AAAI2021 COVID-19 Fake News Detection Shared Task dataset [13], a huge dataset compiled from various origins and meticulously annotated through fact-checking from reputable sources. The fact-checking sources comprise Cable News Network (CNN), World Health Organization (WHO), Centers for Disease Control and Prevention (CDC), Al Jazeera, along with fact-checking websites such as Snopes[1], FactCheck, and Poynter. Table 7.3 shows the proof of fact checking by the above-mentioned sources. Then, the BERT model was created using the PyTorch Pretrained BERT package. The BERT model was fine-tuned using the COVID-19 Fake News dataset and annotated information.

A logistic regression model underwent training to extract insights from the BERT model. Local explanations for predictions were provided using SHAP to enhance user confidence in the condensed BERT model. An experiment involving three conditions – Condition T (Text), Condition TSE (Text+SHAP Explanation), and Condition TSESE (Text+SHAP Explanation+Source and Evidence) – was carried out on Amazon Mechanical Turk[2]. Figure 7.6 (a) shows that participants involved in condition T (namely, Condition 1), were given a COVID-19-related claim and a classifier prediction about whether it was correct or incorrect.

Figure 7.6 (b) depicts the TSE condition (namely, Condition 2) where an explanation using SHAP was furnished alongside the claim and model prediction, aiming to enhance the transparency of the model's predictions. Figure 7.6(c) demonstrates the condition of TSE (namely, Condition 3), where the participants involved in condition

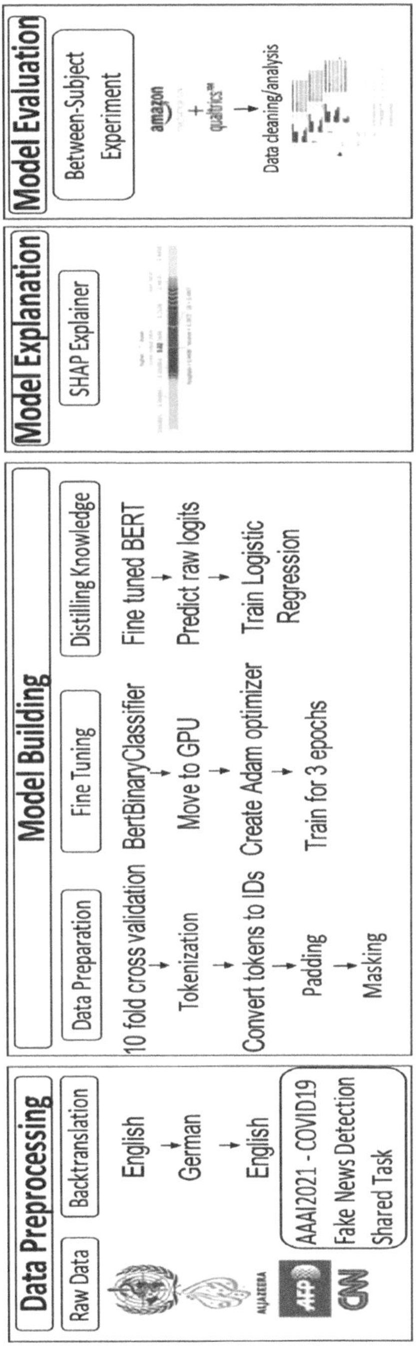


**FIGURE 7.5** DistilBERT using SHAP model [24].

**TABLE 7.3**
**Trustworthy Sources for Fact-checking Claims**

| Label | Source | Date | Claims |
|---|---|---|---|
| Fake | FactCheck | Jan. 28, 2020 | 'Chinese spy team' working in a Canadian government lab sent 'pathogens to the Wuhan facility' prior to the coronavirus outbreak in China. |
| Fake | Snopes | March 2, 2020 | Sales of Corona beer dropped sharply in early 2020 because consumers mistakenly associated the brand name with the new coronavirus. |
| Fake | Poynter | Jan. 22, 2020 | Chinese influencer caused the new coronavirus outbreak after eating bat soup. |
| Fake | WHO | March 20, 2020 | COVID-19 only affects the old. |
| True | CNN | April 9, 2020 | There's no evidence to support the theory that 5G networks cause COVID-19 or contribute to its spread. |
| True | WHO | March 20, 2020 | Being able to hold your breath for 10 s or more without coughing or feeling discomfort DOES NOT mean you are free from COVID-19. |
| True | CDC | April 11, 2020 | Stay home for 14 days after your last contact with a person who has COVID-19. |
| True | FactCheck | March 16, 2020 | Gargling water with salt won't 'eliminate' coronavirus. |

TSESE were given the proof and original source of the allegations. The performance of the proposed model was tested against existing approaches. The proposed method produced significant benefits in identifying COVID-19-related misinformation and in enhancing public confidence.

## 7.5 FAKE NEWS DETECTION USING SOCIAL MEDIA ANALYSIS

Social media are the main source of fake news dissipation. The spread rate of fake news is much faster than any other media due to smartphones and there is no screening mechanism for the validity of posts. The news that spreads is in the form of text, audio, video, or images. Fake news has an impact on a country's economy and politics. Social networks such as Facebook, WhatsApp, X (formerly Twitter), Instagram, and YouTube were the main sources of connection between the people during lockdown. An add-on tool was developed which could be installed in a browser to detect the social networking sites that spread fake information [25].

Researchers have assimilated information about the source of spread which includes name, their profile, site or application, number of users, groups, events, posts, and tags. These data help to analyze and detect the individual and the site or application that spreads the false news. Techniques for analyzing the fake detection include algorithms from NLP, Neural Network, Deep Learning, Machine Learning,

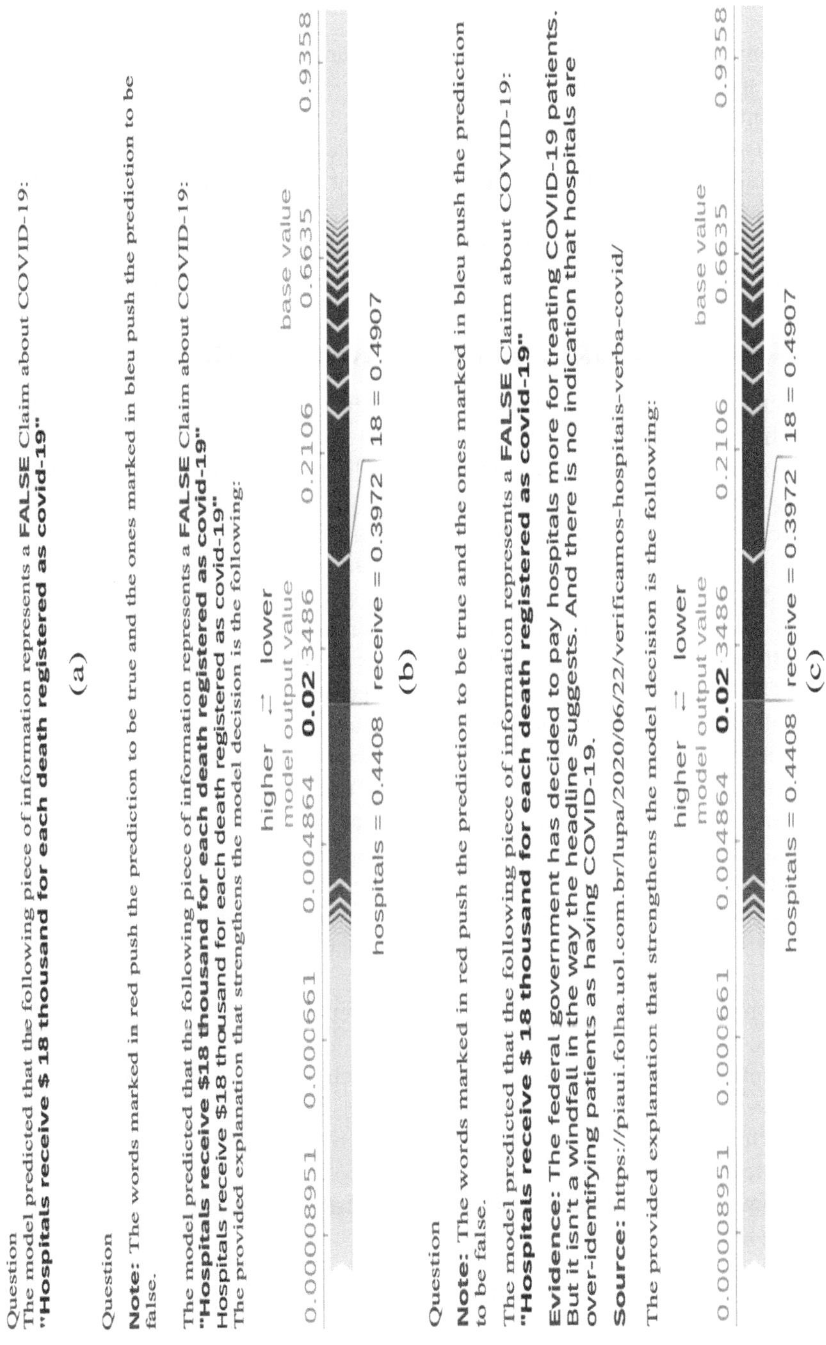


**FIGURE 7.6** Three conditions: (a) Condition 1, (b) Condition 2, and (c) Condition 3 [24].

and Ensemble models to get a tangible solution. Fake news detection techniques focus on the following [2]:

- Identifying the potential users with similar characteristics having common perspectives.
- Identifying malicious accounts.
- Network representations through content analysis and temporal characteristics.
- Social dimension by identifying whether it is posted by humans or robots. Also, time of post and the rate of spread.
- Analysis of terms, language used, and style of content generation.
- Analysis on crowd sourcing, social network traffic, and clickbait.

## 7.6 GRAPH NETWORK FOR FAKE NEWS DETECTION

Several studies were carried out on COVID-19 data related to false news detection. A study from Pakistan was carried out to detect the dissipation of COVID-19 fake news through WhatsApp groups. Data was collected from a valid questionnaire regarding the authenticity of the data forwarded through WhatsApp. Statistical analysis was performed and it revealed that 83.5% of them check the COVID news for authenticity and 63.5% have shown a drastic change in the news reading pattern due to the spread of fake news [5].

Social Network Analysis has a classical approach using graph networks. Griti Gupta (2021) has applied graph network analysis for a Twitter data set for the detection of COVID-19 fake news [3]. Graphical embedding and deep learning techniques were applied for the spread of fake news related to COVID-19 on Twitter. The authors identified the community (social network group) and examined the propagation patterns of genuine and fake news among its users. A Weisfeiler Lehmanc (WL) graph kernel approach was applied to classify graph networks. The WL kernel technique finds the isomorphism between the graphs. It includes node attributes for the classification of graphs without requiring any additional information about the nodes. Different phases of graph classification are represented in Figure 7.7.

The following are approaches in graph classification:

1. From the tweets related to COVID, a dataset with two classes are formed, i.e. fake and true news.
2. Apply the graph generation algorithm, which forms a social network from the tweets.
3. Perform graph embedding and construct a graph model with tweet ID as nodes and the tweet messages as edge.
4. Now, the graph model is ready for classification. Apply the WL kernel technique for classification of nodes.

The study considered 1370 nodes with 1685 edges for genuine news graphs and 863 nodes with 866 edges for fake news graphs. These were used as a model for training the graph classification. From the graph considered for analysis, 39 communities

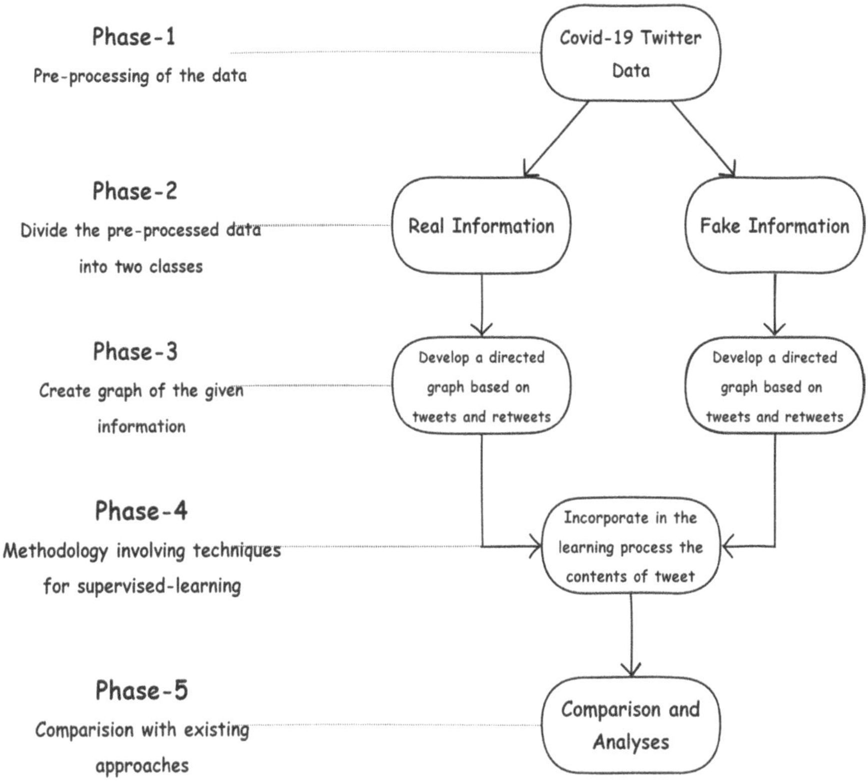


**FIGURE 7.7** Workflow of fake news detection using graph network [3].

were detected as fake, and 60 were considered genuine communities. Density, min, max, and average degree, degree assortativity, degree distribution, and page ranking were considered evaluation metrics for graph analysis.

Graph Neural Network (GNN) is one of the most popular techniques used in Social Network Analysis. GNN represents the characteristics and the properties of the graph through neural network architecture. GNNs are broadly classified as Recurrent Graph Neural Networks, Spatial Convolution Networks, and Spectral convolutional Networks. GNN can be used for the classification of nodes, graphs, and for the prediction of links.

A GNN is constructed with multiple layers of graph that are trained to learn some knowledge from each layer and propagate further to the next level. Figure 7.8 shows the GNN architecture.

GNN can provide a k-hop neighborhood. Each edge, node, and global context in the graph can store information about the graph through edge embedding, vertex embedding, and global embedding. Graphs are represented as adjacency matrices which is the same way of representing pixels of an image. Each node has a different set of neighbors in a graph, unlike images which have a fixed set of neighbors. GNN adopts a graph-in and graph-out model where its input is a graph in which its information is

**FIGURE 7.8** Graph Neural Network representation.

**TABLE 7.4**
**Node Features**

| Feature Class | Feature Name |
|---|---|
| User Based | Is verified user |
| | Number of friends |
| | Number of followers |
| Text Based | Number of hashtags |
| | Number of mentions |
| | Sentiment score computed using VADER |
| | Frequency of positive words |
| Temporal | Frequency of negative words |
| | User account timestamp |
| | Time difference with source node |
| | Time difference with immediate predecessor |
| | Average time difference with the immediate successors |

stored in its nodes, edges, and global context. Its features are represented in Tables 7.4 and 7.5. GNN is the stack of graphs representing the layers. Input and the output layers of GNN are represented with an adjacency matrix that denotes the neighbors in the graph and their relationship. This information about the graph is transferred to subsequent layers of the network without changing the graph structure, i.e. connectivity.

Each layer of the network uses a Multi-Layer Perceptron (MLP) which is applied at every node to learn representation. In this manner, training happens at the node,

**TABLE 7.5**
**Graph Features**

| | |
|---|---|
| num_nodes | Total number of tweets and retweets for a news article |
| num_tweets | Number of tweets |
| avg_num_retweets | Average number of retweets per tweet |
| retweet_perc | Average number of retweets per tweet |
| num_users | Number of unique users |
| total_propagation_time | Amount of time news was referenced on Twitter |
| avg_num_followers | Number of followers averaged over all users |
| avg_num_friends | Number of friends averaged over all users |
| perc_posts_1_hour | Percentage of tweets in first hour of news publish time |
| users_10h | Users reached in 10 hours |
| avg_time_diff | Avg. time between a tweet and its retweet |

edge, and global context level to learn the embedding. Based on the information at the node and edges, predictions can be made. However, it becomes tricky when the edges contain information but the nodes do not. Still a prediction can be performed using the pooling technique. The information is aggregated from each of their embeddings and represented as a matrix. Embeddings can be aggregated using sum, max, or average. For global context prediction, aggregation is applied of all node embeddings using pooling and repeated the same for global edge pooling.

Hamid et al. applied GNN for classifying 5G conspiracy–COVID graph data into three classes: 5G conspiracy, non-conspiracy, and other conspiracy [27]. A four-layered MLP graph architecture was modeled for 5G conspiracy classification. Max and mean functions were applied for neighbor and graph pooling, respectively. The model was trained for 1000 epoch with a 0.01 learning rate and has achieved an AUC of 0.95.

GNN can be used to model complex graphs, capture the linear and non-linear relationships, and can generalize it for test cases. It is one of the best visualization methods for applications. Though GNN is good at modeling, it is very hard to interpret its results, it has complex training algorithms, and it is computationally expensive. Also, it is sensitive to noise and may have overfitting issues.

Some of the popular GNN models used for COVID fake news detection are below.

- Graph Convolution Neural Network (GCN): Architecture has multiple convolution layers to represent the node with quality data.
- Attention-based Graph Neural Network (AGNN): Nodes are represented with aggregate details of the significant neighbors.
- Graph Auto Encoders (GAE): Unsupervised model uses encoding and decoding techniques for node representation using latent information.

Yang (2021) applied GNN on a tweet data set to classify it into fake or real news [28]. Text, Twitter ID, relationship, and other details from social media are extracted

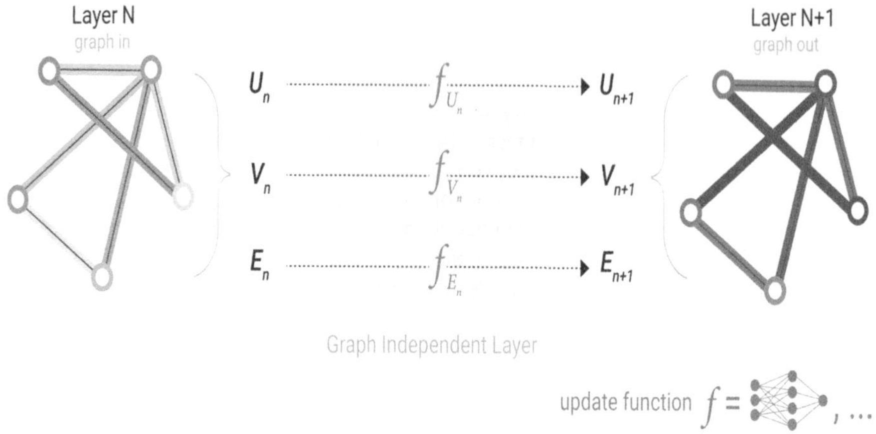


**FIGURE 7.9** Graph Neural Network training [26].

from the source and converted to a text graph. The text graph is applied to GCN to train on semi supervised classification with ReLU as an activation function. The performance of GCN was proven to be superior to the conventional machine learning model even after feature embeddings.

A few attempts were carried out on more than one scheme for fake news prediction. Figure 7.10 shows the architecture of a combined model of content-based and context-based prediction. The context-based model uses a graph network as an input for the model. The content-based model applies on text input. GCN and transfer models are used for training both the inputs, respectively. The results from both the neural network model are concatenated and further processed with a dense network. The output layer is the dense network that classifies the input as fake or real. The variation of this approach is to calculate the class probability from each model. The probabilities of models 1 and 2 are aggregated for prediction [29].

There are many areas as yet untouched by researchers to explore in GNN for constructing a strong model for fake news prediction.

1. Construction of Heterogeneous graph includes text, images, and video features.
2. Dynamic graph construction using real time news data.
3. Multiplex GNN that combines more than one classification scheme like context-based and content-based.

## 7.7 COMBAT THE SPREAD OF FAKE NEWS

As the users of social media, we have to follow a certain etiquette while sharing messages. First, never share or forward information if its source is unknown or not trustworthy. Second, if the information is from one source, then it is susceptible. Real news will be from multiple sources. Thirdly, information is manipulated to make you anxious, emotional, and curious to search further. This emotional hunt makes the user

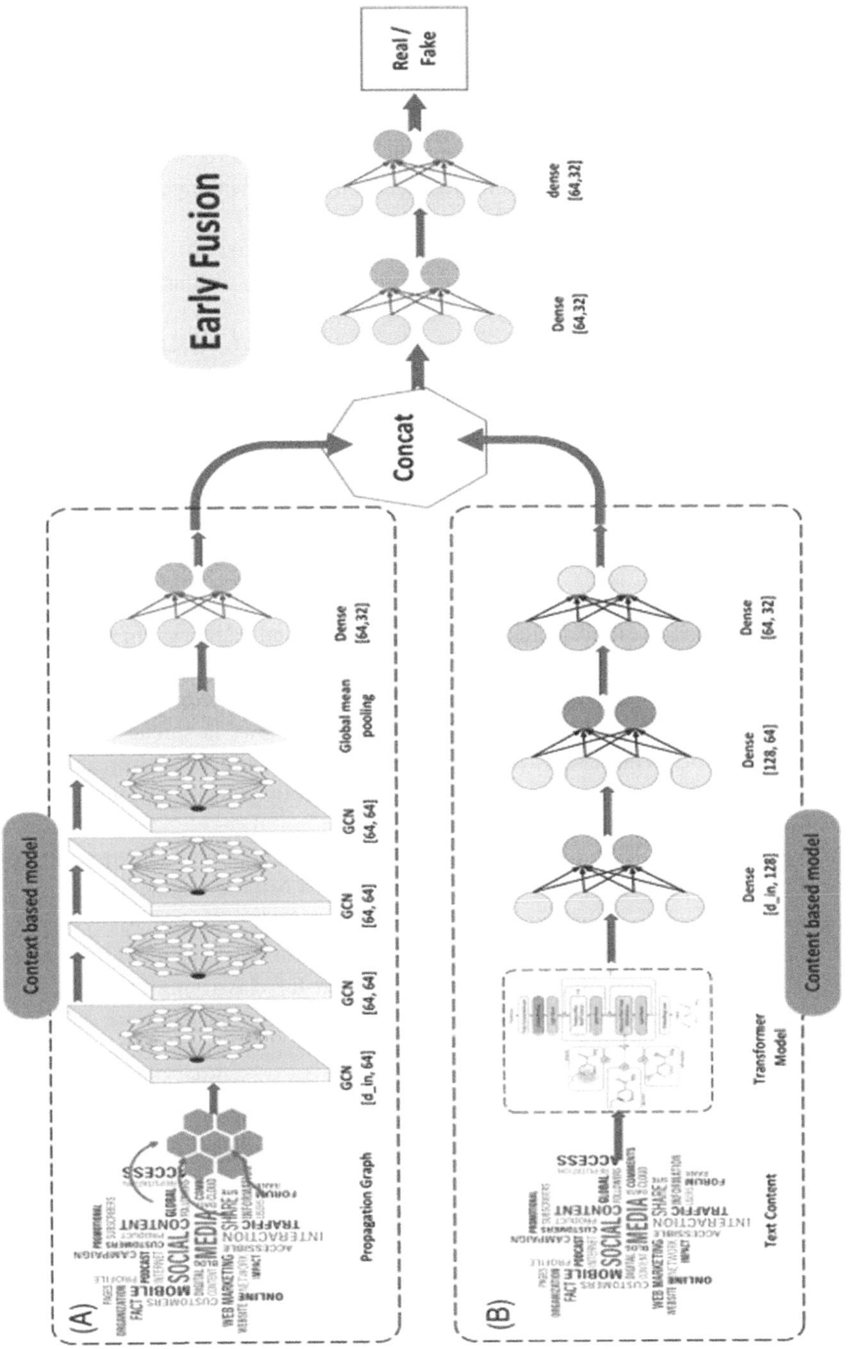


FIGURE 7.10 Multiplex architecture of fake news detection.

go by the misinterpreted or misled facts. Therefore, it is the responsibility of the user to check the validity before sharing the information to a group.

Since, we are in an Artificial Intelligence (AI) era, the spread of fake news can also be done by a bot for an intentional or profit purpose. At the same time, using AI, we can easily identify such bots and prevent the spread of fake news. Websites like Boomlive, Poynter, PolitiFact, and Snopes can be used to validate the authenticity of the news. Many AI techniques can be applied for early detection and mitigation of fake news. Though we are in the fifth generation of AI, challenges still persist for automating the solution to this problem.

1. Benchmark data sets play a crucial role in training algorithms. Graph data sets are not available for analysis.
2. Early fake news detection is the need of the hour. Otherwise, fake news will become 'authentic' and people will start believing it leading to the further spread of fake news.
3. Analysts require sophisticated hardware support to train complex models like GNN for early detection.

## 7.8 CONCLUSION

The spread of fake news is a real challenge in the present world. As lay people, we are not in a position to differentiate easily between fake and real news. In some cases, such as in politics and the stock market, the news can be game changers. The purpose is to gain profit, fame, likes, and subscribers in social media. Fake news can be in the form of text, video, audio, and images. Fake news is spread through the medium of websites, YouTube, X (formerly Twitter), Facebook, WhatsApp, and other social media channels. They actually captivate our emotions to believe and forward the news to others.

Many studies have been carried out over the last decade on the detection of fake news. During the pandemic, the infodemic related to COVID was at its peak

Statistical, Machine Learning, Deep Learning, Social Network Analysis, and Natural Language Processing are the techniques applied for the detection of fake news. Though Machine Learning techniques are well suited for classifying the news, they have limitations with respect to the size of the data. Deep Learning can work on a large volume of data for the supervised and unsupervised application of fake detection. Graph Neural Network techniques can capture the pattern of the spread through the message content as well as the relationship between the users forwarding these messages.

Though researchers have been successful in fake news detection, the work was performed on static data and not on a live stream of news. Some of the other challenges faced are the lack of hardware and computation support to scale up the algorithm and to develop a complex model to suit the need of multifaceted social media data.

## NOTES

1 www.snopes.com
2 www.mturk.com

## REFERENCES


1. Hunt Allcott and Matthew Gentzkow. Social media and fake news in the 2016 election. *Journal of Economic Perspectives*, 31(2):211–236, 2017.
2. Andreea Nistor and Eduard Zadobrischi. The influence of fake news on social media: Analysis and verification of web content during the covid-19 pandemic by advanced ma- chine learning methods and natural language processing. *Sustainability*, 14(17):10466, 2022.
3. Kriti Gupta and Katerina Potika. Fake news analysis and graph classification on a covid- 19 twitter dataset. In *2021 IEEE Seventh International Conference on Big Data Computing Service and Applications (BigDataService)*, pages 60–68. IEEE, 2021.
4. Shankar Biradar, Sunil Saumya, and Arun Chauhan. Combating the infodemic: Covid-19 induced fake news recognition in social media networks. *Complex & Intelligent Systems*, 9(3):2879–2891, 2023.
5. Masroor Ahmed, M Qamar, R Asghar, et al. Fake news shared on whatsapp during covid-19: An analysis of groups and statuses in Pakistan. *Mediaobrazovanie*, 1:4–17, 2021.
6. World Health Organization. COVID-19 Mythbusters – World Health Organization — who.int, 2020. www.who.int/emergencies/diseases/ novel-coronavirus-2019/advice-for-public/myth-busters. [Accessed 03-11-2023].
7. Michael V Bronstein, Gordon Pennycook, Adam Bear, David G Rand, and Tyrone D Cannon. Belief in fake news is associated with delusionality, dogmatism, religious fundamentalism, and reduced analytic thinking. *Journal of Applied Research in Memory and Cognition*, 8(1):108–117, 2019.
8. Kristian G Andersen, Andrew Rambaut, W Ian Lipkin, Edward C Holmes, and Robert F Garry. The proximal origin of sars-cov-2. *Nature Medicine*, 26(4):450–452, 2020.
9. bbcnews. Ofcom: Covid-19 5G theories are 'most common' misinformation — bbc. co.uk. www.bbc.co.uk/news/technology-52370616. [Accessed 03- 11-2023].
10. John Cook, Sander Van Der Linden, Stephan Lewandowsky, and Ullrich KH Ecker. "Coronavirus,'plandemic' and the seven traits of conspiratorial thinking". *The Conversation* 2020. https://theconversation.com/coronavirus-plandemic-and-the-seven-traits-of-conspiratorial-thinking-138483 [Accessed 15-11-2025].
11. Amy Mitchell and J Baxter Oliphant. Americans immersed in covid-19 news; most think media are doing fairly well covering it. 2020.
12. L. Sanders. The difference between what Republicans and Democrats believe to be true about COVID-19. *YouGov,* 2020. https://today.yougov.com/topics/politics/articles-reports/2020/05/26/ republicans-democrats-misinformation. [Accessed 03-11-2023].
13. Huyen Trang Phan, Ngoc Thanh Nguyen, and Dosam Hwang. Fake news detection: A survey of graph neural network methods. *Applied Soft Computing*, 139:110235,2023.
14. Taylor Nelson, Nicole Kagan, Claire Critchlow, Alan Hillard, and Albert Hsu. The danger of misinformation in the covid-19 crisis. *Missouri Medicine*, 117(6):510, 2020.
15. Giselly Mayerly Nieves-Cuervo, Edgar F Manrique-Herna´ndez, Angelo Fernando Robledo-Colonia, and Ardila Elvia Karina Grillo. Infodemic: Fake news and covid-19 mortality trends in six latin american countriesinfodemia: not´ıcias falsas e tendeˆncias na mortalidade por covid-19 em seis pa´ıses da ame´rica latina. *Rev Panam Salud Publica*, 45:e44–e44, 2021.
16. Faizi Fifita, Jordan Smith, Melissa B Hanzsek-Brill, Xiaoyin Li, and Mengshi Zhou. Machine learning-based identifications of covid-19 fake news using biomedical information extraction. *Big Data and Cognitive Computing*, 7(1):46, 2023.

17. Cape Talk. Video claiming Covid-19 tests are contaminated is fake news – WC Health Dept — capetalk.co.za, 2021. www.capetalk.co.za/articles/380006/video-claiming-covid-19-tests-are-contaminated-is-fake-news-wc-health-dept? ref=pid:112. [Accessed 03-11-2023].
18. Afreen Kansal. Fake news detection using POS tagging and machine learning. *Journal of Applied Security Research*, 18(2):164–179, 2023.
19. Carlos Castillo, Marcelo Mendoza, and Barbara Poblete. Information credibility on twitter. In *Proceedings of the 20th International Conference on World Wide Web*, pages 675–684, 2011.
20. Ke Wu, Song Yang, and Kenny Q Zhu. False rumors detection on sina weibo by propagation structures. In *2015 IEEE 31st International Conference on Data Engineering*, pages 651–662. IEEE, 2015.
21. Deepika Varshney and Dinesh Kumar Vishwakarma. An automated multi-web platform voting framework to predict misleading information proliferated during covid-19 outbreak using ensemble method. *Data & Knowledge Engineering*, 143:102103, 2023.
22. Jacob Devlin, Ming-Wei Chang, Kenton Lee, and Kristina Toutanova. Bert: Pre-training of deep bidirectional transformers for language understanding. *arXiv preprint arXiv:1810.04805*, 2018.
23. S Deepak and Bhadrachalam Chitturi. Deep neural approach to fake-news identification. *Procedia Computer Science*, 167:2236–2243, 2020.
24. Jackie Ayoub, X Jessie Yang, and Feng Zhou. Combat covid-19 infodemic using explainable natural language processing models. *Information Processing & Management*, 58(4):102569, 2021.
25. Monther Aldwairi and Ali Alwahedi. Detecting fake news in social media networks. *Procedia Computer Science*, 141:215–222, 2018.
26. Benjamin Sanchez-Lengeling, Emily Reif, Adam Pearce, and Alexander B Wiltschko. A gentle introduction to graph neural networks. *Distill*, 6(9):e33, 2021.
27. Abdullah Hamid, Nasrullah Shiekh, Naina Said, Kashif Ahmad, Asma Gul, Laiq Hassan, and Ala Al-Fuqaha. Fake news detection in social media using graph neural net- works and NLP techniques: A covid-19 use-case. *arXiv preprint arXiv:2012.07517*, 2020.
28. Yuqing Yang. Covid-19 fake news detection via graph neural networks in social media. In *2021 IEEE International Conference on Bioinformatics and Biomedicine (BIBM)*, pages 3178–3180. IEEE, 2021.
29. Pallabi Saikia, Kshitij Gundale, Ankit Jain, Dev Jadeja, Harvi Patel, and Mohendra Roy. Modelling social context for fake news detection: A graph neural network based approach. In *2022 International Joint Conference on Neural Networks (IJCNN)*, pages 01–08. IEEE, 2022.

# 8 Overcoming and Solving the Challenges of Data Deluge in Healthcare

*Anuradha J., B. Venkatesh, and Shivashankar G.*

## 8.1 INTRODUCTION

In this digital era, most sectors, including government organizations, businesses, and individuals, generate large amounts of data, and it keeps growing exponentially. Various sources like websites, digital applications, and devices generate rapid data in real-time, and the data gushes out of the digital medium. This situation leads to a data deluge. Though the analysts are enriched with these data, the success of AI-driven applications lies in how these data are tapped and utilized properly to generate knowledge. Some factors leading to data deluge are technological advancements, social media, user-generated content, the Internet of Things (IoT), business and transactional data, and scientific research and simulations.

The data deluge from various applications may also include invalidated data that needs attention for data engineering. Data engineering aims to investigate and comprehend facts to make wise decisions and create a fresh framework for both practical and cognitive decisions. In the modern world, there are a number of instances of data overload. For instance, social media sites are producing an ever-greater volume of data. Social media users are set to produce 4.4 trillion gigabytes of data in 2022, from which trends can be followed, influences can be found, and marketing initiatives can be targeted using this data. It is challenging to organize and evaluate such massive amounts of data.

Big Data, AI, and data-driven applications have a greater positive impact on society as a whole and various real-life applications of different domains. In contrast, their improper use will be disastrous as it may violate privacy and security concerns. Big Data's 'creep factor' must be addressed immediately, especially due to the availability of the devices at low cost, faster access medium, advancements in internet facility, etc. Society is becoming more 'datafied' as capturing, collecting, storing, and processing data is made easier and simpler. Technological advancement in computational power is a cakewalk for data analysts. In this big data era, every bit of information about our day-to-day activity is recorded by the Government, other organizations, and marketers who can capitalize on it.

An enormous number of IoT devices are available in the market and are easy to use. This has led to a tremendous increase in data generation from sensors, devices, and other interconnected objects [1]. For example, nearly 40 terabytes of data are

DOI: 10.1201/9781003449058-8

generated daily for only a single self-driving car[1]. Social media platforms generate a massive amount of data daily. For example, X (formerly Twitter) and Facebook generate 600 million tweets and 50 billion pieces of content daily. Amazon generates nearly 540 petabytes of data yearly through online transactions. These vast amounts of data create a challenge for organizations and businesses to store, manage, and analyze these data. However, the data deluge also presents an opportunity, as businesses can use this data to gain insights into their customers, operations, and markets.

## 8.2 DATA VOLUME AND ITS TYPES

Businesses are facing challenges due to the volume and diversity of data sources. As digital channels, IoT devices, and social media become more common, data is being generated from various sources and formats. This can make it difficult for businesses to collect, store, and analyze data. Here are some specific challenges that businesses face with data sources [2]:

1. Data volume: The amount of data being generated is growing exponentially, and this is putting a strain on businesses' ability to store and manage it.
2. Data variety: The different types of data that are being generated make it more difficult to organize, manage, and analyze.
3. Data quality: The quality of the data can vary widely, which can make it difficult to get accurate insights.
4. Data security: The data can be vulnerable to cyberattacks, which can have a significant impact on the business.

There are a number of technologies that can help businesses to address the challenges of data sources. These include:

1. Data integration: Data integration can help businesses combine data from different sources into a unified view. This can make it easier to analyze the data and extract insights.
2. Data governance: Data governance can help businesses to ensure that the data is accurate, secure, and compliant with regulations.
3. Data analytics: Data analytics can help businesses to make sense of large volumes of data. This can help them to identify trends, make predictions, and improve decision-making.

By addressing the challenges of data sources, businesses can gain a competitive advantage. They can use the data to improve operations, make better decisions, and develop new products and services.

Data deluge has challenges and opportunities for organizations and businesses to gain valuable insights and make data-driven decisions. But processing, managing, and extracting knowledge from the data requires advanced resources. Organizations have started using big data technologies like Hadoop (distributed storage systems), Spark (data processing frameworks), and Machine Learning (ML) for data analysis and pattern recognition to overcome this. The advancement in AI and ML plays a crucial role in mining knowledge from the vast amount of data that is being generated every day.

### 8.2.1 Challenges

In this subsection, we will address the challenges faced by the data deluge [3].

1. Organizations must spend high operational costs storing vast amounts of data.
2. The data must be protected from data breaches and unauthorized access.
3. As the volume of data increases, we need to compromise on data quality and reliability. Incomplete and noisy data may lead to erroneous decisions.
4. As data is gathered from various sources of different formats, it isn't easy to combine and integrate.
5. In real time, analyzing these large datasets is highly computationally intensive and time consuming. Traditional data processing systems may not be capable of handling the data deluge.
6. Extracting meaningful information from large datasets requires deep domain knowledge and skilled data scientists. There is a shortage of such professionals.
7. Large datasets can inadvertently contain noisy, irrelevant, and redundant data, so which data to discard or retain becomes crucial.
8. Finally, we need some regulatory compliance, such as General Data Protection Regulation (GDPR) [4], to deal with concerns that arise with sensitive data.

Data-driven approaches are adopted by organizations to overcome the challenges of data deluge. It can be achieved by managing, storing, collecting, and analyzing data in such a way that improves the businesses and enables good decision-making. The following are some critical techniques organizations use to overcome challenges.

1. Data prioritization: It focuses on finding and storing valuable and relevant data to the organization's objectives. It helps contribute to crucial business decisions and insights.
2. Data governance: It involves assigning data ownership and access control.
3. Scalable infrastructure: Organizations need flexible and scalable data processing and storage infrastructure such as distributed storage and cloud computing systems for varying data volumes.
4. Big data technologies like Apache Hadoop, Apache Spark, and NoSQL databases are required to efficiently process and analyze large datasets.
5. Real-time data processing requires delivering timely insights from streaming data.
6. To automate the data analysis and identify the hidden patterns in large datasets, techniques such as ML and AI are essential.
7. Eliminate duplicate data to reduce data storage and improve data quality.

By implementing the above-said techniques, organizations can better deal with the data deluge, extract knowledge, and make the correct decisions to improve business outcomes.

The following are some of the fields and industries that are facing the data deluge:

- Healthcare: Electronic health records, IoT sensors
- E-commerce and retail: Online shopping
- Social media: Twitter, LinkedIn
- Financial services: Stock market
- Telecommunication: Mobile phones and internet use
- Industry 4.0: IoT sensors, machine data
- Transportation: GPS tracking
- Energy and utilities: Smart grid data
- Environment monitoring: Weather stations, environmental sensors
- Research and academia: Scientific research
- Media and entertainment: Streaming services
- Marketing and advertising: Digital marketing campaigns
- Smart cities with IoT sensors.

The above-said fields face the data deluge challenge and require advanced data management, storage, and analysis techniques. Data-driven decision-making and insights from this data can lead to innovations, improved services, and increased efficiency across these industries.

## 8.3 DATA DELUGE IN HEALTH CARE

In recent years, extensive research has been seen in healthcare services [5]. Specifically, IoT has shown potential applications in improving the quality of medical services for remote locations. These sensors can be either embedded or wearable on the human body, and they are used in healthcare applications to collect physiological information like pressure rate, electron encephalography (EEG), temperature, heartbeat, blood pressure, electrocardiograph (ECG), and so on [6]. Due to their efficient performance, many IoT devices are being utilized. This is leading to the generation of massive amounts of data. Cloud computing and edge computing are used for quick diagnosis of patients and medical intervention. One efficient solution to overcome the data deluge problem is to build an application that can process this vast amount of data. Statistics [7] show that there will be 1 trillion sensors by 2030, leading to the effective growth of big data technologies.

In [8], the researchers focused on an extensive IoT data survey in the context of how to analyze large amounts of data. The study focused mainly on how researchers put their efforts into analyzing big data, and various big data architectures were proposed for handling data deluge on IoT data.

According to [9], researchers use different types of data analysis for IoT applications. Real-time, offline, memory-level, Business Intelligence (BI), and massive level are the most used types of analytics. Table 8.1 represents the comparative analysis of different analytics at different levels.

**TABLE 8.1**
**Types of Data Analysis in Data Deluge at Various Levels**

| Analytic type | Architecture | Uses | Advantages |
|---|---|---|---|
| Offline [10] | • Time tunnel<br>• Kafka<br>• Scribe | If the response time of applications is highly optional. | • Data format conversion cost is less.<br>• Data acquisition is efficient |
| Real-Time [11] | • HANA<br>• Greenplum | Used to analyze large amounts of data generated by the sensors | Parallel processing of clusters by using traditional DB memory. |
| BI level [12] | Data analysis plans | Apply when the data surpasses the memory level | Both online and offline. |
| Massive level [13] | MapReduce | Apply when the data scale has surpassed the capacity of BI products. | Applicable for offline. |
| Memory level [13] | MongoDB | Apply when the total volume of the data is less than the maximum cluster memory. | Real-time |

In biological science, the data deluge problem has been extensive. Due to technological advancement, genomic sequence data is produced faster and cheaper than to manage, analyze, and store them. To cope with the data flow, most biologists have started using novel approaches that use mathematical tools to find exciting associations in the data.

## 8.4 CHALLENGES OF DATA DELUGE IN A LIFE SCIENCES CONTEXT

The primary challenge in life science data analysis is finding accurate data! There is lots of data available, but it is challenging for scientists to find the interesting data they need. Even though the data is publicly available, even if it is in-house, i.e. a company's private data, the researchers need to understand enough about the context of the data to access and analyze it. Another challenge for the researchers is the sheer volume of data available. How can researchers analyze such vast amounts of data within a reasonable timeframe?

In [14], dealing with the data deluge for microarray data is discussed. According to [14], microarray data collected so far has been generated on multiple platforms and stored in places with different formats, locations, and levels of detail. It makes it very difficult for researchers to group, verify, or analyze the data and compare results with their own. There are no uniform standards for reporting gene data in the journal articles, and they do not require the authors to deposit the data.

## 8.5 NAVIGATING THROUGH A SEA OF INFORMATION

In today's digital age, we are constantly bombarded with overwhelming information. From social media updates to news articles, emails to text messages, we find ourselves swimming in a vast sea of data. Data are valuable assets that can help organizations gain a competitive edge. However, collecting too much data can lead to a data deluge, which can be difficult to manage and secure. Unstructured and unsecured data can also put businesses at risk of privacy and compliance issues.

The average data breach cost in 2022 has climbed to $4.35 million, up 12 percent from 2020. This shows that the cost of data breaches is rising, and businesses must take steps to protect their data.

Here are some tips for managing data deluge and preventing data breaches:

- Only collect the data that we need.
- Keep data organized and secure.
- Use encryption to protect data.
- Train employees in data security best practices.

By following these tips, we can help to protect an organization's data and avoid the costly consequences of data breaches.

1. Only collect the data that we need. This is the most important tip for managing data deluge. If we collect too much data, it will be difficult to manage and secure. Only collect the data needed to run our business and make informed decisions.
2. Keep data organized and secure. Once we have collected the data that we need, we need to keep it organized and secure. This means using a data management system that can help to track and store data. We should also protect data from unauthorized access using different techniques.
3. Use encryption to protect data. Encryption is a way of scrambling data so it cannot be read without a key. This is an important way to protect data from unauthorized access.
4. Train employees in data security best practices. Employees are the first line of defense against data breaches. Make sure that they are trained in data security best practices. This includes things like how to identify phishing emails and how to protect their passwords.

It is also essential for businesses to engage with their customers to ensure that they are aware of how their data is being used and that their privacy is respected. Companies should have a clear and transparent privacy policy that outlines how they use customer data and what measures are in place to protect it. Having a strong understanding of customer preferences and expectations is also a key factor in developing a successful data privacy strategy. By engaging with their customers, businesses can build trust and ensure their data is used responsibly and ethically.

Businesses should also consider developing data analytics capabilities to gain insights from the data they have collected. By leveraging data analytics, companies can gain valuable insights into their customers and the market. This will enable them to make better decisions and develop better strategies for their business. Data analytics also has the potential to enable businesses to better understand their customers, allowing them to deliver more personalized experiences. By utilizing data analytics, businesses can ensure that they are making the most out of the data deluge and maximizing their potential for growth and success. Data breaches can have far-reaching consequences for businesses, including financial penalties, reputational damage, and customer loss. In addition, security risks are constantly evolving, making it difficult for businesses to keep up. Many organizations need more skills and resources to effectively manage data security. This can lead to data breaches, which can have a devastating impact on a business. Here are some of the specific consequences of data breaches.

- Financial penalties: Businesses that suffer data breaches can be fined by regulators. The amount of the fine can be significant, depending on the severity of the breach.
- Reputational damage: Data breaches can damage a business's reputation. Customers may lose trust in the business, and the business may have difficulty attracting new customers.
- Customer loss: Data breaches can lead to customer loss. Customers who have their data compromised may switch to a different business.
- Increased compliance costs: Businesses that suffer data breaches may have to increase their compliance costs. This is because they must implement new security measures to prevent future breaches.

In addition to these direct consequences, data breaches can also have several indirect implications. For example, a data breach can decrease employee productivity, as employees may be worried about their personal data being compromised. Businesses need to take steps to protect their data from breaches. This includes implementing strong security measures like data encryption and access controls. Businesses should also train their employees in data security best practices. By taking steps to protect their data, businesses can help to mitigate the consequences of a data breach.

Decision-makers must take steps to minimize the risk of privacy and compliance breaches. This includes assessing how data is stored and who has access to it. With the right tools, organizations can better manage granular access, auditing, and other processes for maintaining compliance. One way to minimize the risk of privacy and compliance breaches is to use the cloud. Cloud vendors handle data backups and shoulder much of the security burden. This can free decision-makers to focus on other aspects of their business, such as innovation and growth. Here are some specific steps that decision-makers can take to minimize the risk of privacy and compliance breaches:

- Assess how data is stored and who has access to it: This includes identifying all of the data stored in the organization and who has access to it.

- Implement strong security measures, including data encryption, access controls, and auditing.
- Train employees on data security best practices: This includes things like how to identify phishing emails and how to protect their passwords.
- Use the cloud: Cloud vendors handle data backups and shoulder much of the security burden.

By taking these steps, decision-makers can help to minimize the risk of privacy and compliance breaches.

## 8.6 CLOUD FOR DATA HANDLING

Software-as-a-service (SaaS) solutions are a good fit for organizations that can provide cloud services for data storage and processing. This is because SaaS solutions are scalable and elastic, which means that they can be easily scaled up or down to meet the needs of the organization. In addition, SaaS solutions are often more secure than on-premises systems. This is because cloud providers have invested heavily in security, and they have the expertise to keep data safe. As technologies like IoT, tools with distributed workforces, and social media proliferate, they create data for organizations that need an efficient way to securely leverage those data. The cloud offers several advantages over on-premises systems in this regard. For example, the cloud can provide the following benefits for data deluge.

- Scalability: The cloud can be easily scaled up or down to meet the needs of the organization. This is important for organizations that need to be able to handle spikes in traffic or data volume.
- Security: Cloud providers have invested heavily in security and have the expertise to keep data safe. This is important for organizations that need to protect sensitive data.
- Cost-effectiveness: The cloud can be a cost-effective way to store and manage data. This is because cloud providers can spread the cost of infrastructure across multiple organizations.

As a result, it is not surprising that nearly 70% of IT decision-makers say their companies have hastened moves to the cloud during the past year. The cloud offers a number of advantages over on-premises systems, and it is becoming the preferred way to manage content and data.

## 8.7 DATA DELUGE IN IOT

Most medical analysis has been carried out with IoT sensors in recent years due to technological advancement. As many patients and individuals use these Healthcare IoT (HIOT) sensors, a massive amount of data is generated. Acquiring, integrating, storing, processing, and using these data have become important problems for enterprises to achieve their business goals. A cloud computing platform helps with processing, storing, and analyzing IoT data. As these sensor devices produce massive amounts of heterogeneous data, it is challenging to handle it for analysis. The characteristics of IoT data in cloud platforms are summarized as follows [15].

- Multisource High Heterogeneity Data
- Huge Scale Dynamic Data
- Low-Level with weak Semantic Data
- Inaccuracy Data

An IoT application framework [16] consists of three layers: perception, network, and application. In a cloud computing environment, the application layer is critical for IoT-based storage systems; it comprises middleware and business models.

Figure 8.1 shows the detailed role of each layer in the IoT-based framework for data storage in the cloud. The framework consists of many modules, such as:

- Data acquisition and integration: This module, used as the input, deals with acquiring and integrating heterogeneous data from various sensor devices.
- Data storage: The data acquired from different sensors will be in structured, unstructured, and semi-structured formats. Different DB or file systems are required to handle these: XML files for HDFS, RDBMS, and NoSQL.
- Management: Approaches like data index, metadata, semantic relations, and linked data are used for the efficient retrieval of data from large volumes of sources, with the best efficiency.

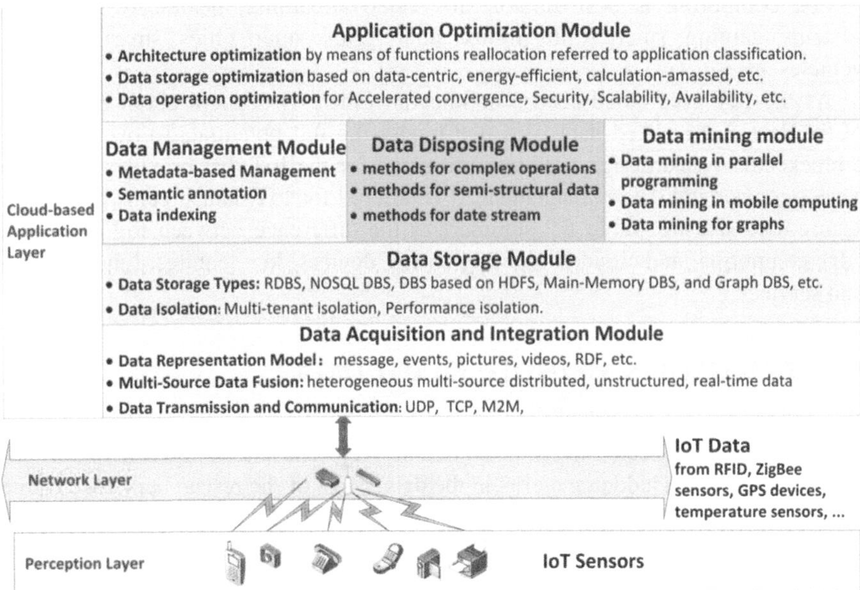


**FIGURE 8.1** Framework of IoT-based data storage systems in cloud computing [16].

- Processing: MapReduce is constructed for parallel and distributed data processing of massive data.
- Mining: The data extracted from sensors are always raw and low-level data; data mining is required to extract a high level of data from the IoT data to achieve comprehensive views for end users.
- Application optimization: Different performance requirements are needed depending on the analysis of applications and algorithms required for processing IoT data in the cloud platform. Such as ad security, scalability, management, decreased costs and prices, etc.

The existing Cloud Computing (CC) uses hash algorithms as IoT data access storage algorithms but has a low fault tolerance rate and processing efficiency. To overcome this, Hadoop Distributed File System (HDFS) [17] has been introduced to optimize IoT CC data access storage algorithms. Hash values maximize the configuration of data access storage distribution in the IoT. IoT data is currently processed in the cloud, and the computing environment is distant from the sensors. Consequently, N/W bandwidth and communication latency become severe bottlenecks. Edge computing was introduced to overcome issues related to network congestion and computing delay [18, 19] by processing data as close as possible to sensors or directly on user devices. Muhammad Rizwan Anawar et al. [20] proposed a systematic review of IoT data computing using fog computing. Fog computing is a replacement for edge computing, where the computing of the IoT data happens near the sensor devices to overcome the latency problem faced in cloud computing. In fog computing, the computing is done by creating a micro cloud (fog nodes) at the proximity edge of data sources.

Fog computing is best suitable for video streaming, healthcare monitoring systems, gaming, smart traffic lights, smart grids, smart cities, smart connected vehicles, etc.

As the IoT uses cloud-centric architecture, there is concern about the security of the data, i.e. isolated data silos that hinder the full potential. To overcome this, a blockchain-based design [21] was presented for the IoT that provides distributed access control and data management. It is tailored for IoT data streams and enables secure data sharing. Table 8.2 summarizes the difference between fog computing, edge computing, and cloud computing on IoT devices' key features, functionalities, and services.

## 8.8 EVALUATION METHODS OF IOT DATA

The following section will discuss the different evaluation techniques available to process the data collected from the sensor devices. These techniques help decision-making and extract hidden patterns in the data. Most of the researchers use Machine Learning (ML) and Deep Learning (DL) algorithms for making decisions [22]. Generally, most researchers use a standard workflow model consisting of collecting the data, analysis of data, visualizing data, and evaluating data [23]. Figure 8.2 represents the workflow model for IoT data.

**TABLE 8.2**
**Fog vs Cloud vs Edge Computing**

| Features | FOG computing | Edge computing | Cloud computing |
|---|---|---|---|
| **Availability of server nodes** | Availability high range of servers | Less scalable than fog computing | Availability of a few servers |
| **Type of services** | Distributed and localized, limited and special for a specific domain | Mainly used in cellular mobile networks | Worldwide and global services |
| **Location identification** | Yes | Yes | No |
| **Mobility features** | Provided and fully supported | Provided and partially supported | Limited |
| **Real-time interaction** | Supported | Supported | Supported |
| **Real-time response** | Highest | Higher | Lower |
| **Ample data storage and duration** | Short duration and targeted to a specific area | It depends on the scenario of services and applications | Lifetime duration as its managing big data |
| **Big data analytic capacity and computation quality** | Short-time capacity with high-level computation functionality | Short time capacity for prioritized computing facilities | Long-time capacity only with categorization computing facilities |
| **Working environment and positions** | Streets, roadside, homes, malls, field tracks (e.g., every Internet existing area) | Deployed by the specific services provider in specific indoor areas | Indoors with massive components at a cloud service provider-owned place |
| **Architectural design** | Distributed | Distributed | Centralized |
| **The number of users facilitated** | Locally related fields (e.g., IoT, STL devices) | Specific related areas (e.g., mobile users) | General Internet-connected users |
| **Major service provided** | Cisco IOx, Intel | Cellular network companies | Google, Amazon, IBM, and Microsoft Azure |

Source: [20].

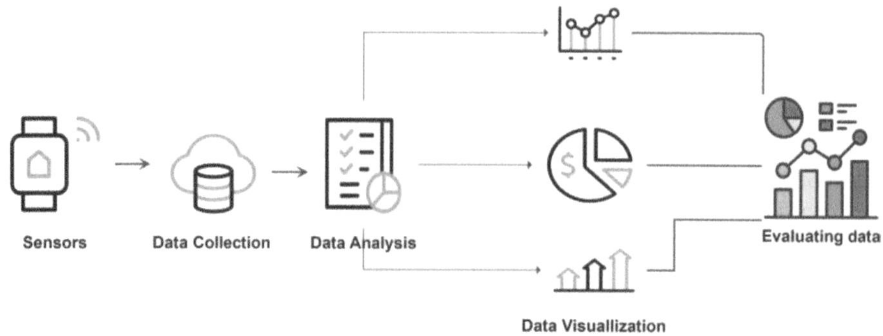


**FIGURE 8.2** Workflow model for IoT data.

Out of the workflows, data analysis plays a crucial role in using ML algorithms to train the model with historical data. The model performs data visualization, and evaluation is carried out for unseen data. ML algorithms are available for various generated data types, such as classifying data with class labels and clustering for data without target attributes. Popular classification algorithms such as logistic regression, Support Vector Machine (SVM), and Random Forest are used for datasets to decide whether a person is affected by a specific disease. In contrast, regression algorithms are used for problems such as traffic condition forecasting [24], tracking vehicles [25], estimating delivery time [26], etc.

As the number of devices connected to the internet increases, the data collected also increases. To analyze such colossal data, standard algorithms are essential. So, to cope with the increase in data volume, deep learning algorithms are required for efficient data evaluation. Bolhasani et al. [27] presented a systematic review of deep learning applications in the IoT and healthcare domain. Figure 8.3 represents a comprehensive classification of the DL IoT applications in healthcare.

Based on the study by McKinsey on the IoT global economic consequences [28], the annual economic effect of IoT in 2025 will range from $2.7 to $6.2 trillion. About 41% of the most significant share is from the healthcare sector, followed by 33% and 7% by industry and oil, respectively. And the remaining percentage is from irrigation, transport, public infrastructure, security, and retailers of the entire IoT sector.

Zhao et al. [29] provided a systematic overview of DL research on IoT for healthcare by machine. Four aspects of DL architecture are reported in Auto-encoder models, the Restricted Boltzmann model, CNN, and RNN. Tuli et al. [30] proposed Health Fog for the diagnosis of heart diseases automatically using DL and IoT. Fog services perform fast processes on the acquired data and reduce network latency. Faust et al. [31] proposed a DL model based on LSTM using heart rate signals to detect atrial fibrillation (AF) episodes. To evaluate the performance of the proposed model the MIT-BIH Atrial Fibrillation Dataset was used. The proposed model achieved 98.51% accuracy with 10-fold cross-validation.

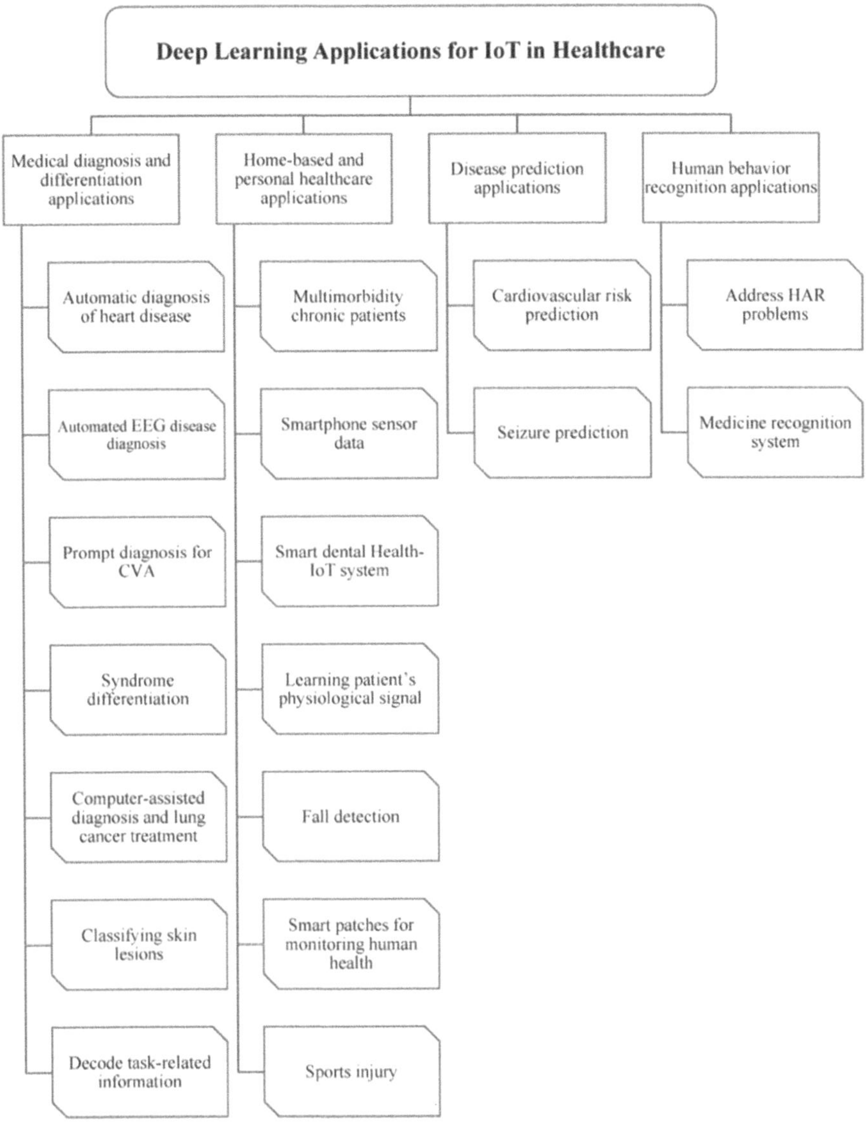


**FIGURE 8.3** Taxonomy of deep learning applications for IoT in healthcare [27].

Bray et al. [32] proposed a computer-assisted diagnosis for lung cancer treatment using a deep reinforcement learning model. The proposed model can spot lung tumors and predict a valid outcome.

Ma and Tavares [33] proposed a model to identify skin cancer using IoT technology. The proposed model can identify melanoma as a severe skin cancer caused by metastasis. Generally, melanocytic lesions are of one three types: melanomas, common nevi, and atypical nevi.

## 8.9 ADAPTING TO THE DATA DELUGE

Overcoming the data deluge in healthcare requires a combination of strategic planning, technological solutions, and data management best practices. Here are some effective strategies to manage and make the most of the large volumes of data generated in the healthcare domain.

- Comprehensive data strategy: Develop a comprehensive data strategy that outlines clear goals, data governance policies, data security measures, and data quality standards. This strategy should align with the organization's overall objectives and support data-driven decision-making.
- Data governance and privacy: Implement robust data governance practices to ensure data is properly collected, stored, and used. Adhere to data privacy regulations such as HIPAA (in the United States) or GDPR (in the European Union) to protect patient information.
- Cloud-based solutions: Leverage cloud computing and storage services to handle the scalability demands of healthcare data. Cloud solutions offer cost-effective and scalable options for managing large datasets while ensuring data security and accessibility.
- Advanced analytics and machine learning: Utilize advanced analytics and machine learning algorithms to efficiently process and analyze healthcare data. These technologies can help derive meaningful insights, identify patterns, and predict outcomes.
- Data standardization and interoperability: Establish data standardization and interoperability frameworks to facilitate seamless data exchange between different healthcare systems, devices, and institutions. This enables a comprehensive view of patient data and enhances collaboration.
- Real-time data processing: Implement real-time data processing capabilities to handle streaming data from wearable devices, sensors, and monitoring systems. This enables timely clinical interventions and decision-making.
- Data compression and archiving: Use data compression techniques to reduce storage space requirements, especially for medical imaging data. Consider archiving older or less frequently accessed data to optimize storage resources.
- Data retention policies: Establish data retention policies that define how long data should be stored and when it can be securely deleted or archived. This prevents unnecessary accumulation of data and reduces storage costs.
- Collaboration and partnerships: Collaborate with external partners, re- search institutions, and data experts to share expertise, resources, and datasets. Collaborative efforts can lead to better insights and research outcomes.
- Data literacy and training: Invest in data literacy training for healthcare professionals and staff. Educate them on the importance of data privacy, security, and effective use of data analytics tools to support evidence-based decision-making.
- Automated data cleaning and validation: Implement automated data cleaning and validation processes to ensure data accuracy and reliability. This reduces errors in the data and enhances data quality.

- Security and privacy measures: Deploy robust cybersecurity measures to safeguard healthcare data from potential breaches and cyberattacks. Regularly update security protocols to stay ahead of evolving threats.
- Focus on value: Prioritize data initiatives that deliver tangible value to patients, healthcare providers, and the organization. Focus on projects that improve patient outcomes, care coordination, and operational efficiencies.

By adopting these strategies, healthcare organizations can navigate the data deluge effectively, harness the power of data-driven insights, and enhance patient care while ensuring data security and privacy. A well-structured approach to data management empowers healthcare professionals to make informed decisions, innovate healthcare practices, and contribute to advancements in medical research and population health management.

## 8.10 GUIDE FOR DECISION-MAKERS

An example of a data deluge in healthcare is the proliferation of medical imaging data. Medical imaging technologies, such as X-rays, CT scans, MRIs, ultrasounds, and digital pathology slides, produce a massive amount of data for each patient study. As these technologies advance, the volume and resolution of medical images continue to increase, leading to a data deluge in healthcare.

1. Increasing volume of medical images: Advancements in medical imaging technologies have significantly increased the number of medical images produced for each patient study. For instance, a single CT scan may consist of hundreds of cross-sectional images, while an MRI study can generate thousands of images, capturing detailed views of different body structures. Multiply this by the number of patients undergoing imaging studies daily, and healthcare organizations are faced with an overwhelming amount of image data.
2. High-resolution and 3D imaging: Modern medical imaging devices pro- duce images with higher resolution and three-dimensional capabilities. Higher resolution images result in finer details, which are crucial for accurate diagnoses. Additionally, 3D imaging allows for a more comprehensive view of anatomical structures, which aids in surgical planning and treatment decisions. However, these advancements also contribute to the data deluge, as each image contains more data points and requires larger storage space.
3. Multiple imaging modalities: In addition to traditional X-rays, healthcare providers use a variety of imaging modalities, such as computed tomography (CT), magnetic resonance imaging (MRI), ultrasounds, and digital pathology. Each modality generates its own set of images and data. Integrating and managing these diverse data sources pose challenges for healthcare organizations.
4. Repeat studies and follow-ups: In clinical practice, patients may undergo multiple imaging studies over time for different medical conditions, disease

monitoring, or follow-up examinations. These repeat studies generate redundant data, further contributing to the data deluge.

5. Research and population studies: Medical imaging data is essential not only for individual patient care but also for medical research and population studies. Research projects involving large cohorts of participants and multiple imaging sessions generate vast amounts of data for analysis and insights.
6. Data storage and management challenges: Storing and managing the massive volume of medical imaging data require substantial storage capacity and efficient data management systems. Healthcare organizations must invest in robust, scalable infrastructure to handle the data load.
7. Data analysis complexity: Analyzing and processing medical images is computationally intensive and time-consuming, especially when dealing with large datasets. Advanced image processing and machine learning algorithms are employed to extract valuable information from the images.
8. Data sharing and collaboration: Medical imaging data is valuable for collaborative research and multidisciplinary care. However, securely sharing and exchanging large medical image files while complying with patient privacy regulations can be challenging.
9. Interoperability and standardization: To fully utilize medical imaging data, it is essential to establish interoperability standards that allow seamless data exchange between different healthcare systems and imaging devices. Standardization efforts, such as the Digital Imaging and Communications in Medicine (DICOM) standard, aim to address this challenge.

To address the data deluge in medical imaging, healthcare providers are increasingly adopting cloud-based storage and processing solutions. Cloud computing offers the scalability and resources needed to store, manage, and analyze large volumes of medical images efficiently. Moreover, cloud-based solutions support secure data sharing, collaboration, and remote access, enabling healthcare organizations to leverage imaging data effectively for improved patient care and medical research.

- Identify trends in patient health data. By analyzing large datasets of patient health data, healthcare organizations can identify trends in diseases, treatments, and outcomes. This information can be used to improve the quality of care and make better decisions about resource allocation.
- Develop personalized treatment plans. By combining patient health data with data from other sources, such as environmental and genetic data, healthcare organizations can develop personalized patient treatment plans. This can lead to better patient outcomes and reduce the cost of care.
- Improve the efficiency of healthcare operations. By analyzing data from electronic health records (EHRs), healthcare organizations can identify areas where operations can be improved. This can lead to reduced costs and improved patient satisfaction.

- Detect fraud and abuse. By analyzing billing data, healthcare organizations can detect fraud and abuse. This can help to protect patients and ensure that healthcare dollars are used appropriately.

## 8.11 RECOMMENDATIONS

The data deluge is a result of organizations collecting more data and the advancement of technology. This data can be a valuable asset for any business' decision-making. However, if decision-makers are able to keep up with the pace of data collection and analysis, the value of the data can be recovered. The data deluge presents challenges and opportunities for various industries, including healthcare. Here are some key takeaways related to the data deluge:

- Vast data growth: The data deluge is characterized by an exponential increase in the volume of data generated, collected, and stored across different sectors. It is driven by technological advancements, the digitization of information, and the proliferation of connected devices. Big data technologies and cloud services support data volume.
- Storage and processing challenges: Dealing with enormous datasets requires significant storage capacity and computational power. Organizations must invest in robust infrastructure and technologies to efficiently manage and process large volumes of data. Distributed techniques for storage and processing are yet another solution for the storage and comprehension of data.
- Opportunities for insights: Amidst the data deluge, there are valuable insights and knowledge hidden within the data. Extracting meaningful information through advanced analytics, machine learning, and data mining can bring significant discoveries and business advantages.
- Data quality and veracity: As data volumes grow, ensuring data quality and accuracy becomes increasingly crucial. Proper data governance, validation processes, and data cleansing are essential to maintain data integrity and reliability.
- Real-time processing: Some applications demand real-time data processing and analysis. Organizations must employ technologies that can handle streaming data and make informed decisions in real time.
- Data privacy and security: With large datasets come increased risks of data breaches and privacy violations. Protecting sensitive information is of the utmost importance, and organizations must implement robust security measures and comply with data privacy regulations. Techniques such as federated learning (FL) will serve this purpose.
- Interoperability and integration: The data deluge often results in data silos, hindering seamless integration and collaboration. Establishing interoperability standards and data exchange mechanisms is essential to unlock the full potential of data.
- Data governance and ethics: As data becomes more pervasive, ethical considerations surrounding data use, ownership, and consent become critical.

Organizations must adopt responsible data governance practices and adhere to ethical guidelines.

- Resource optimization: Organizations must optimize their data management processes to reduce costs, improve efficiency, and make data-driven decisions. Data engineering will provide clean and compact data ready for processing.
- Innovation and transformation: The data deluge encourages organizations to innovate and transform their operations. By leveraging data analytics, artificial intelligence, and other emerging technologies, businesses can gain a competitive edge and adapt to changing market dynamics.
- Collaboration and partnerships: Collaborating with external partners and data experts can help organizations leverage diverse datasets and gain fresh insights, leading to better decision-making.
- Data literacy and skill development: With the influx of data, there is a growing demand for individuals with data literacy and analytical skills. Investing in workforce training and development is crucial to making the most of the data deluge.
- Regulatory compliance: As data regulations evolve, organizations must stay informed about data-related laws and comply with the relevant legal requirements to avoid penalties and reputational damage.
- Sustainability and environmental impact: As data storage and processing consume significant energy resources, organizations should consider sustainable practices to minimize their environmental footprint.
- Navigating the data deluge effectively requires a comprehensive and strategic approach. Organizations must be agile, innovative, and responsible in managing data while focusing on extracting actionable insights that drive positive outcomes for businesses and society as a whole.

## 8.12 CONCLUSION

Data is pouring out from various digital media, which has grabbed the attention of researchers to invest, plan, and organize the data. Data can enrich knowledge, but at the same time, it is hazardous when mishandled. Serious concerns with regard to the data deluge are the variety of data, rate of data flow, its format, varied storage, access methods, security, and privacy. Big data technology enables analysts to store and process data in a distributed and hassle-free manner. It also enables the analyst to work on the live data stream. Federated learning works on individual handheld de- vices by preserving privacy and security for data kept on local devices without being shared with the server. It constructs a distributed model on local devices and builds a global model from the local updates. Thus, a global model is constructed by imbibing knowledge from different local devices. This makes a convenient platform for handling data with ease. Data engineering is another direction that provides efficient methods for cleaning, reducing, and formatting data for analysis. Data privacy is yet another important direction of focus in a data deluge. Mishandled data may cause serious problems for an individual in many ways. As digital advancement creates a hard time with the data deluge, technological development provides an easy and simple solution for every problem faced due to the data deluge. Standardized policies, good practices, and recommendations followed in data creation, handling, and use will be a boon for knowledge engineering and AI-based expert systems. The objectives of the data analyst will be met if AI applications are safe and secure to use, and at the same time, data should not be a burden for the device to store and process.

## NOTE

1 www.forbes.com/sites/forbestechcouncil/2022/02/14/autonomous-vehicles-and-their-impact-on-the-economy/?sh=1644e9fb60de

## REFERENCES


1. Sabyasachi Dash, Sushil Kumar Shakyawar, Mohit Sharma, and Sandeep Kaushik. Big data in healthcare: Management, analysis and future prospects. *Journal of Big Data*, 6(1):1–25, 2019.
2. Simon Elias Bibri and John Krogstie. The big data deluge for transforming the knowledge of smart sustainable cities: A data mining framework for urban analytics. In *Proceedings of the 3rd International Conference on Smart City Applications*, pages 1–10, 2018.
3. Karima Kourtit, Peter Elmlund, and Peter Nijkamp. The urban data deluge: Challenges for smart urban planning in the third data revolution. *International Journal of Urban Sciences*, 24(4):445–461, 2020.
4. Chris Jay Hoofnagle, Bart Van Der Sloot, and Frederik Zuiderveen Borgesius. The European union general data protection regulation: What it is and what it means. *Information & Communications Technology Law*, 28(1):65–98, 2019.
5. Bikash Pradhan, Saugat Bhattacharyya, and Kunal Pal. Iot-based applications in health- care devices. *Journal of Healthcare Engineering*, 2021:1–18, 2021.
6. Haipeng Peng, Ye Tian, Ju¨rgen Kurths, Lixiang Li, Yixian Yang, and Daoshun Wang. Secure and energy-efficient data transmission system based on chaotic compressive sensing in body-to-body networks. *IEEE Transactions on Biomedical Circuits and Systems*, 11(3):558–573, 2017.
7. Min Chen, Shiwen Mao, Yin Zhang, Victor CM Leung, et al. *Big data: Related technologies, challenges and future prospects*, volume 100. Springer, 2014.
8. Mohsen Marjani, Fariza Nasaruddin, Abdullah Gani, Ahmad Karim, Ibrahim Abaker Targio Hashem, Aisha Siddiqa, and Ibrar Yaqoob. Big iot data analytics: Architecture, opportunities, and open research challenges. *IEEE Access*, 5:5247–5261, 2017.
9. CL Philip Chen and Chun-Yang Zhang. Data-intensive applications, challenges, techniques and technologies: A survey on big data. *Information Sciences*, 275:314–347, 2014.
10. Ming Cheng, Wenyan Jia, Xiaorong Gao, Shangkai Gao, and Fusheng Yang. Mu rhythm-based cursor control: An offline analysis. *Clinical Neurophysiology*, 115(4):745–751,2004.
11. Michael W Pfaffl. A new mathematical model for relative quantification in real-time RT–PCR. *Nucleic Acids Research*, 29(9):e45–e45, 2001.
12. Zack Jourdan, R Kelly Rainer, and Thomas E Marshall. Business intelligence: An analysis of the literature. *Information Systems Management*, 25(2):121–131, 2008.

13. Albert Bifet, Geoff Holmes, Bernhard Pfahringer, Philipp Kranen, Hardy Kremer, Timm Jansen, and Thomas Seidl. Moa: Massive online analysis, a framework for stream classification and clustering. In *Proceedings of the first Workshop on Applications of Pattern Analysis*, pages 44–50. PMLR, 2010.
14. Diane Gershon. Dealing with the data deluge. *Nature*, 416(6883):889–891, 2002.
15. Hongming Cai, Boyi Xu, Lihong Jiang, and Athanasios V Vasilakos. IoT-based big data storage systems in cloud computing: Perspectives and challenges. *IEEE Internet of Things Journal*, 4(1):75–87, 2016.
16. Mohammad Aazam, Imran Khan, Aymen Abdullah Alsaffar, and Eui-Nam Huh. Cloud of things: Integrating internet of things and cloud computing and the issues involved. In *Proceedings of 2014 11th International Bhurban Conference on Applied Sciences & Technology (IBCAST) Islamabad, Pakistan, 14th-18th January, 2014*, pages 414–419. IEEE, 2014.
17. Mingzhe Wang and Qiuliang Zhang. Optimized data storage algorithm of iot based on cloud computing in distributed system. *Computer Communications*, 157:124–131, 2020.
18. Gopika Premsankar, Mario Di Francesco, and Tarik Taleb. Edge computing for the internet of things: A case study. *IEEE Internet of Things Journal*, 5(2):1275–1284, 2018.
19. Olivier Debauche, Sa¨ıd Mahmoudi, and Adriano Guttadauria. A new edge computing architecture for iot and multimedia data management. *Information*, 13(2):89, 2022.
20. Muhammad Rizwan Anawar, ShangguangWang, Muhammad Azam Zia, Ahmer Khan Jadoon, Umair Akram, Salman Raza, et al. Fog computing: An overview of big iot data analytics. *Wireless Communications and Mobile Computing*, 2018:715192, 2018.
21. Hossein Shafagh, Lukas Burkhalter, Anwar Hithnawi, and Simon Duquennoy. Towards blockchain-based auditable storage and sharing of iot data. In *Proceedings of the 2017 on Cloud Computing Security Workshop*, pages 45–50, 2017.
22. Kuruva Lakshmanna, Rajesh Kaluri, Nagaraja Gundluru, Zamil S Alzamil, Dharmendra Singh Rajput, Arfat Ahmad Khan, Mohd Anul Haq, and Ahmed Alhussen. A review on deep learning techniques for iot data. *Electronics*, 11(10):1604, 2022.
23. Tao Huang, Liang Lan, Xuexian Fang, Peng An, Junxia Min, and Fudi Wang. Promises and challenges of big data computing in health sciences. *Big Data Research*, 2(1):2–11, 2015.
24. Manoel Castro-Neto, Young-Seon Jeong, Myong-Kee Jeong, and Lee D Han. Online-SVR for short-term traffic flow prediction under typical and atypical traffic conditions. *Expert Systems with Applications*, 36(3):6164–6173, 2009.
25. Sandy Mahfouz, Farah Mourad-Chehade, Paul Honeine, Joumana Farah, and Hichem Snoussi. Target tracking using machine learning and Kalman filter in wireless sensor networks. *IEEE Sensors Journal*, 14(10):3715–3725, 2014.
26. Fangxin Wang, Yifei Zhu, FengWang, Jiangchuan Liu, Xiaoqiang Ma, and Xiaoyi Fan. Car4pac: Last mile parcel delivery through intelligent car trip sharing. *IEEE Transactions on Intelligent Transportation Systems*, 21(10):4410–4424, 2019.
27. H Bolhasani, M Mohseni, and AM Rahmani. Deep learning applications for IoT in health care: A systematic review. *Informatics in Medicine Unlocked*, 23(march):100550, 2021.
28. James Manyika, Michael Chui, Jacques Bughin, Richard Dobbs, Peter Bisson, and Alex Marrs. *Disruptive technologies: Advances that will transform life, business, and the global economy*, volume 180. McKinsey Global Institute, 2013.

29. Rui Zhao, Ruqiang Yan, Zhenghua Chen, Kezhi Mao, Peng Wang, and Robert X Gao. Deep learning and its applications to machine health monitoring. *Mechanical Systems and Signal Processing*, 115:213–237, 2019.
30. Shreshth Tuli, Nipam Basumatary, Sukhpal Singh Gill, MohsenKahani, Rajesh Chand Arya, Gurpreet SinghWander, and Rajkumar Buyya. Healthfog: An ensemble deep learning based smart healthcare system for automatic diagnosis of heart diseases in integrated iot and fog computing environments. *Future Generation Computer Systems*, 104:187–200, 2020.
31. Oliver Faust, Alex Shenfield, Murtadha Kareem, Tan Ru San, Hamido Fujita, and U Rajendra Acharya. Automated detection of atrial fibrillation using long short-term memory network with RR interval signals. *Computers in Biology and Medicine*, 102:327–335, 2018.
32. Hyuna Sung, Jacques Ferlay, Rebecca L Siegel, Mathieu Laversanne, Isabelle Soerjomataram, Ahmedin Jemal, and Freddie Bray. Global cancer statistics 2020: Globocan estimates of incidence and mortality worldwide for 36 cancers in 185 countries. *CA: A Cancer Journal for Clinicians*, 71(3):209–249, 2021.
33. Zhen Ma and Joa˜o Manuel RS Tavares. A novel approach to segment skin lesions in dermoscopic images based on a deformable model. *IEEE Journal of Biomedical and Health Informatics*, 20(2):615–623, 2015.

# 9 Utilizing Artificial Intelligence for the Identification of Plant Species and Detection of Diseases through Deep Learning

*Usha Divakarla, K. Chandrasekaran, Srihari Govindarajan, and Sivaramakrishnan Sangameswaran*

## 9.1 INTRODUCTION

An automated system for identifying plant species and diagnosing diseases could significantly benefit both botanists and individuals with limited botanical knowledge by rapidly providing accurate identifications. Deep learning proves robust in feature extraction, offering enhanced insights into image details. In this study, leaf images underwent preprocessing, and a Convolutional Neural Network (CNN) was employed for feature extraction. In order to increase accuracy, adaptability, and training efficiency, the study presents a mathematical framework for the identification and diagnosis of plant diseases using deep learning techniques.

A dataset of sick leaves placed on a simple background is used to train a transfer learning model with segmented leaf input. After that, the model is tested for rust illnesses, bacterial plaque, and black rot. CNN is used to categorize plant diseases, and the model' s importance is demonstrated via histogram approaches. The diagnosis of pepper leaf diseases is made easier by integrating GoogleNet into a basic CNN architecture. The model's performance is illustrated graphically through training and validation accuracy, and its evaluation in both Color and Grey Scale modes is based on the F1-score.

Image processing finds various applications in agriculture, encompassing the identification of diseased leaves, stems, or fruits, measurement of the affected area by diseases, and determination of the color of the affected region. In India, tomato cultivation stands out as a highly profitable agricultural venture. The conventional method of visual inspection by experts is time-consuming, especially in vast farms or expansive land areas.

 DOI: 10.1201/9781003449058-9

Utilizing image processing techniques for the early detection and identification of tomato plant diseases can significantly enhance product quality. These systems monitor the plant, focusing on features such as leaves and stems. Any deviations from characteristic features are automatically identified, and notifications are promptly relayed to the user, streamlining the detection and notification process.

## 9.2 LITERATURE SURVEY

The author in [1] introduces methods for classifying and detecting plant leaf diseases. The process involves pre-processing steps before feature extraction. Initially, RGB images are transformed into white, then further converted into grey-level images to extract the vein image from each leaf. Subsequently, basic morphological functions are applied to the image, followed by its conversion into a binary image. If a binary pixel has a value of 0, it is converted to the corresponding RGB image value. Finally, disease detection is carried out using Pearson correlation, Dominating feature set, and a Naïve Bayesian classifier.

The process outlined by the author in [2] comprises four steps. The initial step involves collecting images from various regions of the country for both training and testing purposes. In the second phase, a Gaussian filter is employed to eliminate noise, and thresholding is applied to isolate the all-green color component. Segmentation is carried out using K-means clustering. Additionally, all RGB images are converted into HSV to facilitate feature extraction.

The article [3] introduces a method for identifying diseases in jute plants through image processing. The process involves capturing an image and adjusting its size to match the database storage requirements. Subsequently, the image undergoes quality enhancement, and noise removal is performed. Hue-based segmentation is applied to the image using a customized thresholding formula. Further, the image is converted from RGB to HSV to facilitate the extraction of the region of interest. This proposed approach proves particularly beneficial in detecting diseases that affect the stems of jute plants.

According to the study presented in paper [4], the proposed technique aims to detect diseases in paddy plants by comparing them with 100 healthy images, 100 samples of disease1, and another 100 samples of disease2. However, the method acknowledges that merely having training data is insufficient for effective disease detection or classification, particularly when the training data is not linearly separable.

In the research outlined in paper [5], the process for identifying unhealthy plant leaves involves several steps. This includes acquiring an RGB image, converting it from RGB to HSI format, masking, and removing green pixels. The components are then segmented using Otsu's method, texture features are computed using the color-co-occurrence methodology, and finally, disease classification is carried out using a Genetic Algorithm.

In the investigation described in paper [6], tomato disease detection is achieved through computer vision. Initially, a grayscale image is transformed into a binary image based on a threshold value, with the segmentation relying on a threshold algorithm. However, recognizing the limitations of thresholding, particularly in distinguishing ripe and unripe tomatoes, the study introduces the K-means clustering algorithm to overcome these drawbacks. This numerical, unsupervised, nondeterministic, and iterative method creates a specific number of non-hierarchical clusters. The infected parts are then separated from the leaf, and the RGB image is converted into YcbCr to enhance image features. The final step involves calculating the percentage of infection and distinguishing between ripe and unripe tomatoes.

The methodology for detecting cucumber diseases is outlined in paper [7]. This approach encompasses image acquisition, image pre-processing, feature extraction utilizing the grey level co-occurrence matrix (GLCM), and eventual classification through two methods: unsupervised classification and supervised classification. It's important to note that the paddy plant holds significance in continental regions.

In paper [8], RGB images undergo conversion into grayscale using color conversion. Image quality enhancement involves employing various techniques such as histogram equalization and contrast adjustment. The study utilizes different classification features, including SVM, ANN, and FUZZY classification. Feature extraction incorporates diverse feature values such as texture, structure, and geometric features. Utilizing ANN and FUZZY classification, the system is capable of identifying diseases in paddy plants.

## 9.3 PROPOSED SYSTEM

The proposed system has an end-to-end Android application with TFLite that detects plant diseases [9] [10]. It has the algorithms and models to recognize species and diseases in the crop leaves by using a Convolutional Neural Network [11]. The proposed system uses Collab to edit source code. The Plant Village dataset contains 54,305 images of plant leaves (both diseased and healthy) obtained under controlled imaging conditions. The Plant Village dataset comprises 54,305 images of diseased and healthy plant leaves collected under controlled conditions. The images cover 14 species of crops, including: apple, lady's finger, grape, orange, peach, pepper, potato, brinjal, strawberry, and tomato.

### 9.3.1 System Architecture

The design phase diagram and the data flow diagram of the proposed system are illustrated in Figure 9.1 and Figure 9.2, respectively.

To evaluate the effectiveness of our methods on novel, unseen data and to monitor the potential for overfitting in any approach, we conducted experiments using various train-test set splits, such as the 80–20 split. The Plant Village dataset comprises multiple images of the same leaf captured from different angles, with mappings available for 41,112 out of the 54,306 images. Throughout these train-test splits, we ensured exclusive assignment of all images of the same leaf to either the training or testing set. In each experiment, we calculated mean precision, mean recall, mean F1 score, and overall accuracy at regular intervals during training (at the end of each epoch). The final mean F1 score served as the basis for comparing results across different experimental configurations. Our evaluation centered on the suitability of deep

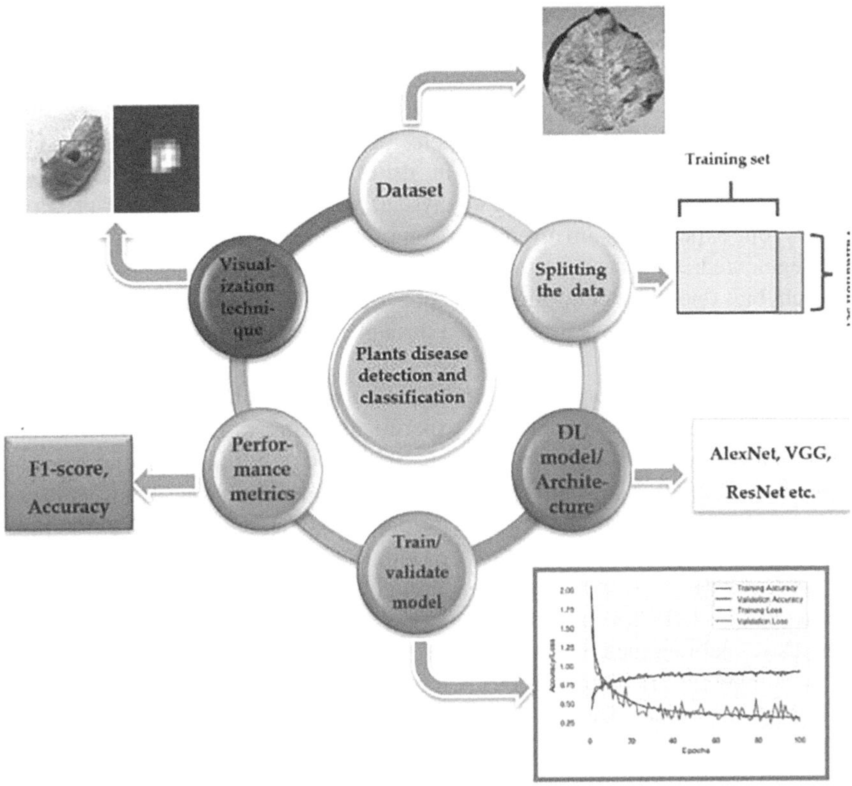


**FIGURE 9.1** Design phase diagram.

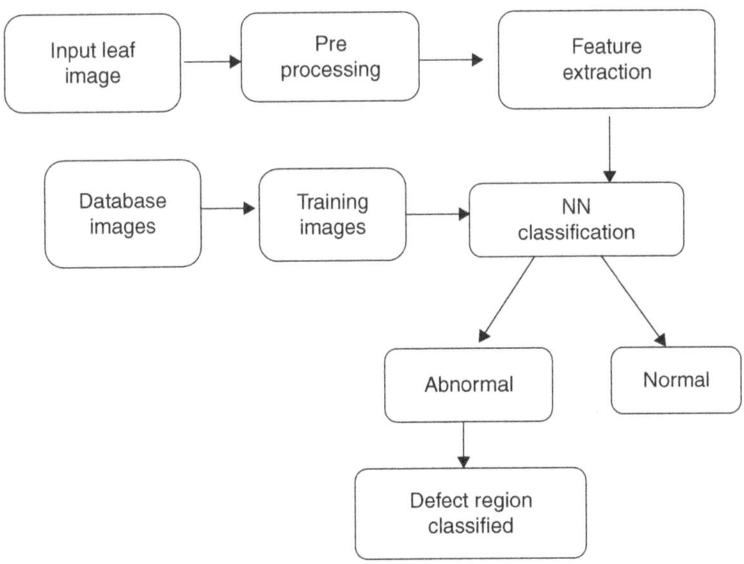


**FIGURE 9.2** Data flow diagram.

convolutional neural networks for the specified classification problem, with a particular emphasis on the GoogleNet architecture. In contrast to the shallower AlexNet, GoogleNet is a more extensive architecture with 22 layers but a significantly lower parameter count (5 million) in the network.

All experiments utilize three versions of the complete Plant Village dataset. Initially, we employed the dataset in its original color format. Subsequently, experiments were conducted using a grayscale variation of the Plant Village dataset. Finally, our experiments involved a version of the Plant Village dataset where leaves are segmented, eliminating excess background information that might introduce inherent bias due to the controlled data collection process in the Plant Village dataset. The segmentation process is automated through a script tailored to perform well on our specific dataset [12].

To assess the effectiveness of our methods on new and unseen data and to monitor the risk of overfitting, we conducted experiments using various train-test set splits, with a particular focus on an 80–20 split. The GoogleNet architecture, in contrast to the less complex AlexNet, is both deeper and wider, featuring 22 layers but with a considerably lower parameter count (5 million) compared to AlexNet (60 million parameters). A noteworthy aspect of the GoogleNet architecture is the incorporation of the 'network in network' concept through inception modules . These modules utilize parallel 1x1, 3x3, and 5x5 convolutions along with a max-pooling layer simultaneously, enabling the concurrent capture of diverse features. To manage computational complexity, 1x1 convolutions before and after the 3x3, 5x5 convolutions (and after the max-pooling layer) are included for dimensionality reduction. The outputs of these parallel layers are concatenated in a filter concatenation layer, forming a single inception module. Our experiments involve the utilization of a total of nine inception modules in the GoogleNet architecture.

The performance evaluation of both architectures on the Plant Village dataset includes training the model from scratch in one scenario and adapting pre-trained models (originally trained on the ImageNet dataset) through transfer learning in another scenario. In transfer learning, we re-initialize the weights of specific layers in both AlexNet and GoogleNet. Throughout training, there are no constraints on the learning of any layers, distinguishing the transfer learning approach from training from scratch. The key difference lies in the initial state of weights for certain layers, enabling the transfer learning approach to leverage visual knowledge acquired by pre-trained models from ImageNet.

## 9.4 IMPLEMENTATION

### 9.4.1 Algorithm

- Input the image into the convolution layer.
- Select parameters and apply filters with strides, incorporating padding if necessary.
- Conduct convolution on the image, followed by the application of ReLU (Rectified Linear Unit) activation to the resulting matrix.

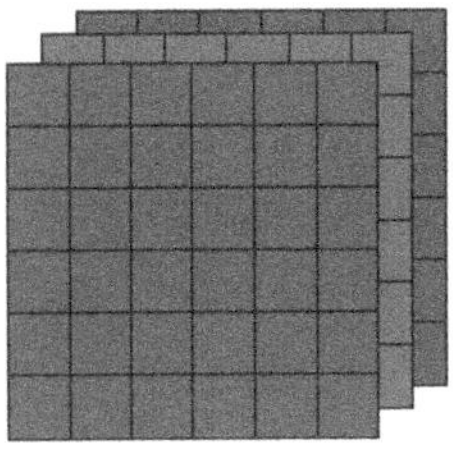


**FIGURE 9.3** RGB matrix (6 x 6 x 3).

- Implement pooling to reduce the size of dimensionality.
- Repeat the process by adding convolutional layers as needed.
- Flatten the output and input it into a fully connected layer (FC Layer).
- Output the class using an activation function, such as Logistic Regression with cost functions, thereby classifying images.

### 9.4.2 Explanation

Convolutional Neural Network (CNN) image classification involves taking an input image, processing it, and categorizing it into specific classes (such as Healthy leaf, Bacterial spot, Late blight, Curl virus, etc.). From the computer's perspective, an input image is perceived as an array of pixels, with its structure depending on the image resolution, denoted as h x w x d (where h = Height, w = Width, and d = Dimension). For example, an image may be represented as a 6 x 6 x 3 array of matrices for RGB values, as illustrated in Figure 9.3, or a 4 x 4 x 1 array of matrices for a grayscale image.

In the process of training and testing a deep learning CNN model, each input image undergoes a sequence of convolution layers with filters (kernels), pooling, fully connected layers (FC Layers), and the application of the SoftMax function to classify an object with probabilistic values ranging between 0 and 1.

### 9.4.3 Convolution Layer

The initial layer in the process, convolution serves to extract features from the input image. This operation maintains the pixel relationships by identifying image features through small squares of input data. It is a mathematical operation involving two inputs: the image matrix with dimensions h x w x d and a filter or kernel matrix with dimensions fh x fw x d. The output is a matrix with dimensions (h – fh + 1) x (w – fw + 1) x 1. An example of a convolutional 3*3 matrix is shown in Figure 9.4.

#### 9.4.3.1 Strides

Stride refers to the quantity of pixel shifts across the input matrix. In cases where the stride is set to 1, the filters move one pixel at a time. Conversely, with a stride of 2, the filters shift by 2 pixels at each step, and this pattern continues. The process of convolution with a stride of 2 is illustrated in Figure 9.5.

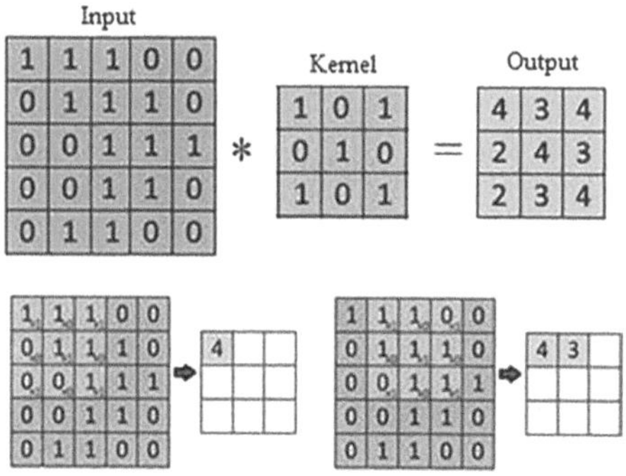


FIGURE 9.4 Convolutional matrix (3 x 3).

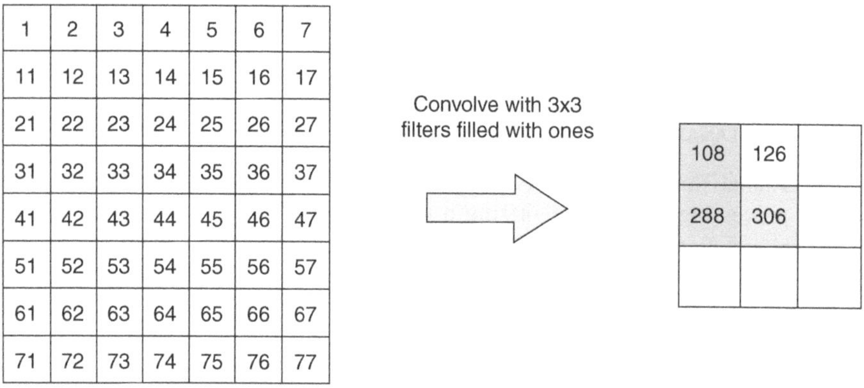


FIGURE 9.5 A stride of 2 pixels.

### 9.4.4 Padding

In situations where the filter does not align perfectly with the input image, there are two available options:

- Zero-pad the image, adding zeros to ensure a proper fit.
- Omit the portion of the image where the filter does not align. This approach is known as valid padding, retaining only the valid section of the image.

#### 9.4.4.1 Non-Linearity (ReLU)

ReLU stands for Rectified Linear Unit for a non-linear operation. The output is $f(x) = \max(0, x)$.

#### 9.4.4.2 Max Pooling

Pooling layers section would reduce the number of parameters when the images are too large. Max pooling takes the largest element from the rectified feature map as shown in Figure 9.6.

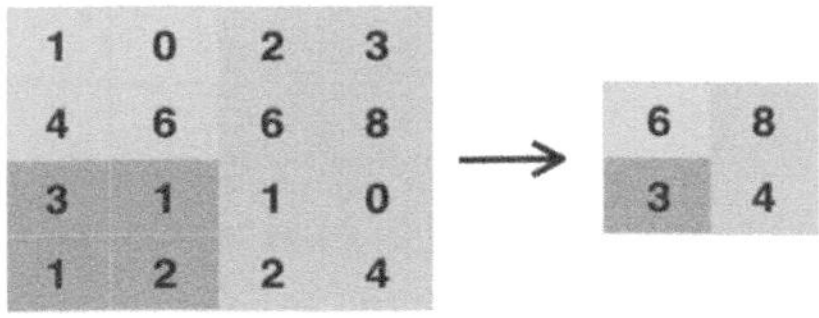


**FIGURE 9.6** An example of max pooling.

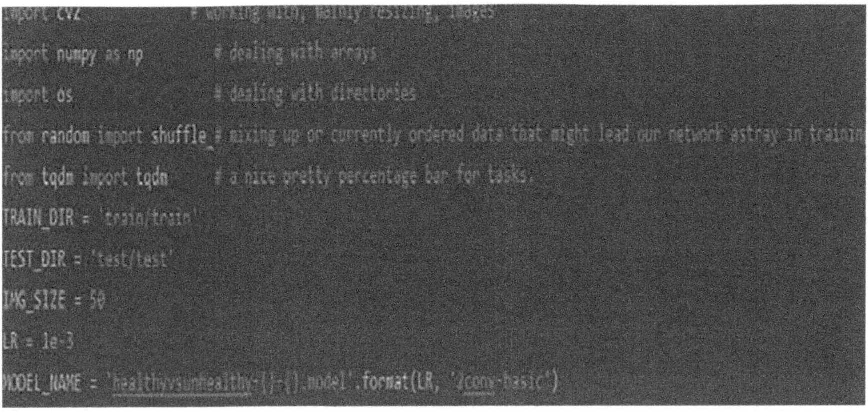

```
import cv2                 # working with, mainly resizing, images
import numpy as np         # dealing with arrays
import os                  # dealing with directories
from random import shuffle # mixing up or currently ordered data that might lead our network astray in trainin
from tqdm import tqdm      # a nice pretty percentage bar for tasks.
TRAIN_DIR = 'train/train'
TEST_DIR = 'test/test'
IMG_SIZE = 50
LR = 1e-3
MODEL_NAME = 'healthyvsunhealthy-{}-{}.model'.format(LR, '2conv-basic')
```

**FIGURE 9.7** Code snippet for importing and setting constants for pre-processing.

## 9.5 CODE SNIPPETS

### 9.5.1 CNN.PY

We possess the data, but it's not feasible to directly input raw images into our convolutional neural network. Initially, we must ensure that all images share the same size, and it's likely that we'll prefer to standardize them to RGB format. TensorFlow Fold simplifies the implementation of deep-learning models designed to handle data with diverse sizes and structures. To begin with, we'll set up our imports and constants for the preprocessing, as depicted in Figure 9.7.

Now, our first order of business is to convert the images and labels to array information that we can pass through our network. To do this, we'll need a helper function to convert the image name to an array. We also build another function to fully process the training images and their labels into arrays as demonstrated in the functions present in Figure 9.8.

The tqdm module is a really nice, pretty way to measure where you are in a process, rather than printing things out at intervals etc., it gives a progress bar.

In any case, the aforementioned function handles the conversion of data into an array format comprising the image and its corresponding label. Once all the images have been processed, we perform a shuffle and subsequently save the data. Since the shuffle operation modifies a variable in place, there is no need to redefine it here.

This function serves the dual purpose of saving the array data and returning it. This approach allows for efficiency when making changes solely to the neural

```
def label_img(img):
    word_label = img[0]

    if word_label == 'h': return [1,0,0,0]

    elif word_label == 'b': return [0,1,0,0]
    elif word_label == 'v': return [0,0,1,0]
    elif word_label == 'l': return [0,0,0,1]

def create_train_data():
    training_data = []
    for img in tqdm(os.listdir(TRAIN_DIR)):
        label = label_img(img)
        path = os.path.join(TRAIN_DIR,img)
        img = cv2.imread(path,cv2.IMREAD_COLOR)
        img = cv2.resize(img, (IMG_SIZE,IMG_SIZE))
        training_data.append([np.array(img),np.array(label)])
    shuffle(training_data)
    np.save('train_data.npy', training_data)
    return training_data
```

**FIGURE 9.8** Code snippet for processing images and their labels.

network's structure without affecting the images, such as alterations in image size. In such cases, we can simply load the array file, saving on processing time. Additionally, a function (see Figure 9.9) is created to process the testing data, which lacks labels. Subsequently, we can initiate the training process using the code outlined in Figure 9.10.

Next, we're ready to define our neural network and we need to reset the graph instance, since we're doing this in a continuous environment, as shown in Figure 9.11

What we have here is a nice, two-layered convolutional neural network, with a fully connected layer, and then the output layer. First, we just want to see how 3 epochs trains, but then, after 3, maybe we're done, or maybe we want to see about 5 epochs. We want to be saving our model after every session, and reloading it if we have a saved version, so we added see Figure 9.12). Next, we split the training and testing data (see Figure 9.13).

Currently, both the training and testing data sets are labeled datasets. The training data will be utilized to train the neural network, while the test data will serve for result validation. The test data is considered "out of sample," indicating that it will solely be employed to assess the accuracy of the network, not for its training.

Additionally, we possess images labeled as "test" that were downloaded. These images lack any labels. The process of creating our data arrays is illustrated in Figure 9.14, following which we proceed to train for 8 epochs (refer to Figure 9.15).

```
def process_test_data():
    testing_data = []
    for img in tqdm(os.listdir(TEST_DIR)):
        path = os.path.join(TEST_DIR,img)
        img_num = img.split('.')[0]
        img = cv2.imread(path,cv2.IMREAD_COLOR)
        img = cv2.resize(img, (IMG_SIZE,IMG_SIZE))
        testing_data.append([np.array(img), img_num])

    shuffle(testing_data)
    np.save('test_data.npy', testing_data)
    return testing_data
```

**FIGURE 9.9** Code snippet for processing test data.

```
train_data = create_train_data()
# If you have already created the dataset:
train_data = np.load('train_data.npy')
```

**FIGURE 9.10** Code snippet for training the model.

Now, since we are happy with the accuracy retrieved from our model, we'll go ahead and save the model.

### 9.5.2 UI.PY

Moving on to the user interface section of our project, we have ui.py. We import the packages shown in Figure 9.16 to create a window-based UI. After which, we deploy a window titled PLANT DISEASE DETECTION (see Figure 9.17).

We now begin to create separate windows using tkinter to display the remedies for the specific diseases that are identified. We start off with the bacterial spot remedies (Figure 9.18), followed by the remedies for the yellow leaf curl virus that are

```
import tflearn
from tflearn.layers.conv import conv_2d, max_pool_2d
from tflearn.layers.core import input_data, dropout, fully_connected
from tflearn.layers.estimator import regression
import tensorflow as tf
tf.reset_default_graph()

convnet = input_data(shape=[None, IMG_SIZE, IMG_SIZE, 3], name='input')

convnet = conv_2d(convnet, 32, 3, activation='relu')
convnet = max_pool_2d(convnet, 3)

convnet = conv_2d(convnet, 64, 3, activation='relu')
convnet = max_pool_2d(convnet, 3)

convnet = conv_2d(convnet, 128, 3, activation='relu')
convnet = max_pool_2d(convnet, 3)

convnet = conv_2d(convnet, 32, 3, activation='relu')
convnet = max_pool_2d(convnet, 3)

convnet = conv_2d(convnet, 64, 3, activation='relu')
convnet = max_pool_2d(convnet, 3)

convnet = fully_connected(convnet, 1024, activation='relu')
convnet = dropout(convnet, 0.8)

convnet = fully_connected(convnet, 4, activation='softmax')
convnet = regression(convnet, optimizer='adam', learning_rate=LR, loss='categorical_crossentropy', name='target

model = tflearn.DNN(convnet, tensorboard_dir='log')
#tensorboard --logdir=log
```

**FIGURE 9.11** Code snippet for defining the neural network.

```
f os.path.exists('{}.meta'.format(MODEL_NAME)):
    model.load(MODEL_NAME)
    print('model loaded!')
```

**FIGURE 9.12** Code snippet for saving and reloading the model.

```
train = train_data[:-500]
test = train_data[-500:]
```

**FIGURE 9.13** Code snippet for splitting the data.

```
X = np.array([i[0] for i in train]).reshape(-1,IMG_SIZE,IMG_SIZE,3)
Y = [i[1] for i in train]

test_x = np.array([i[0] for i in test]).reshape(-1,IMG_SIZE,IMG_SIZE,3)
test_y = [i[1] for i in test]
```

**FIGURE 9.14** Code snippet for creating the data arrays.

```
model.fit({'input': X}, {'targets': Y}, n_epoch=8, validation_set=({'input': test_x}, {'targets': test_y}),
    snapshot_step=40, show_metric=True, run_id=MODEL_NAME)
```

**FIGURE 9.15** Code snippet for fitting the data.

```
import tkinter as tk
from tkinter.filedialog import askopenfilename
import shutil
import os
import sys
from PIL import Image, ImageTk
```

**FIGURE 9.16** Code snippet for importing packages used in creating the User Interface (UI).

```
indow = tk.Tk()

indow.title("PLANT DISEASE DETECTION")

indow.geometry("500x550")
indow.configure(background = "gray")

itle = tk.Label(text=" Click below to choose picture for testing disease", background = 'gray', fg="black", font=("", 15))
itle.grid()
```

**FIGURE 9.17** Code snippet for creating the UI window.

```
ef bact():
    window.destroy()
    window1 = tk.Tk()

    window1.title("PLANT DISEASE DETECTION")

    window1.geometry("600x370")
    window1.configure(background="gray")

    def exit():
        window1.destroy()
    rem = "The remedies for Bacterial Spot are:\n\n "
    remedies = tk.Label(text=rem, background="black",
                        fg="White", font=("", 15))
    remedies.grid(column=0, row=5, padx=10, pady=10)
    rem1 = " Discard or destroy any affected plants. \n  Do not compost them. \n  " \
           "Rotate your plants yearly to prevent re-infection next year. \n Use copper fungicite
    remedies1 = tk.Label(text=rem1, background="gray",
                         fg="Black", font=("", 12))
    remedies1.grid(column=0, row=8, padx=10, pady=10)

    button = tk.Button(text="Exit", command=exit)
    button.grid(column=0, row=9, padx=20, pady=20)

    window1.mainloop()
```

**FIGURE 9.18** Code snippet for creating the window for Bacterial Spot Remedies.

displayed very subtly (Figure 9.19), and the last window is designed for Late Blight Disease on plants (Figure 9.20).

The code snippets (see Figures 9.21 and 9.22) show the implementation for testing of the test image. The image provided can be any of the following classes:

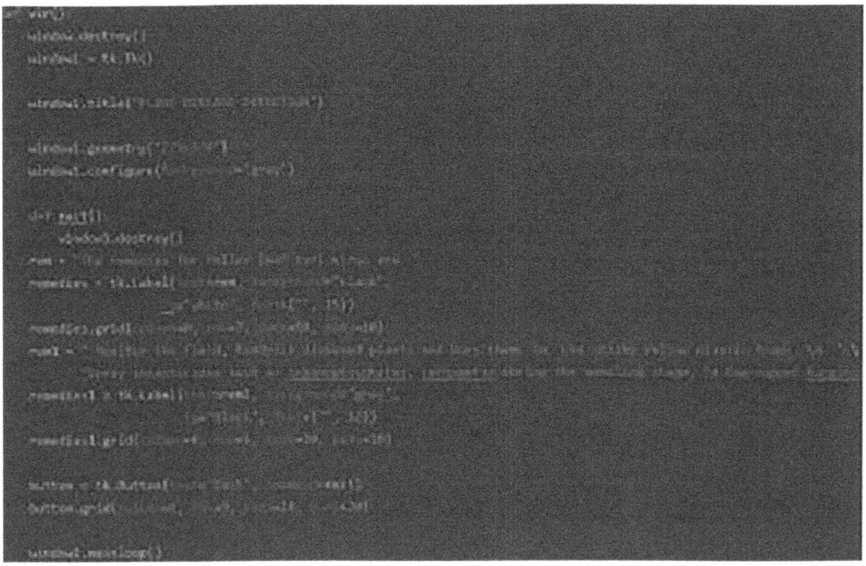

**FIGURE 9.19** Code snippet for creating the window for Yellow Leaf Curl Virus.

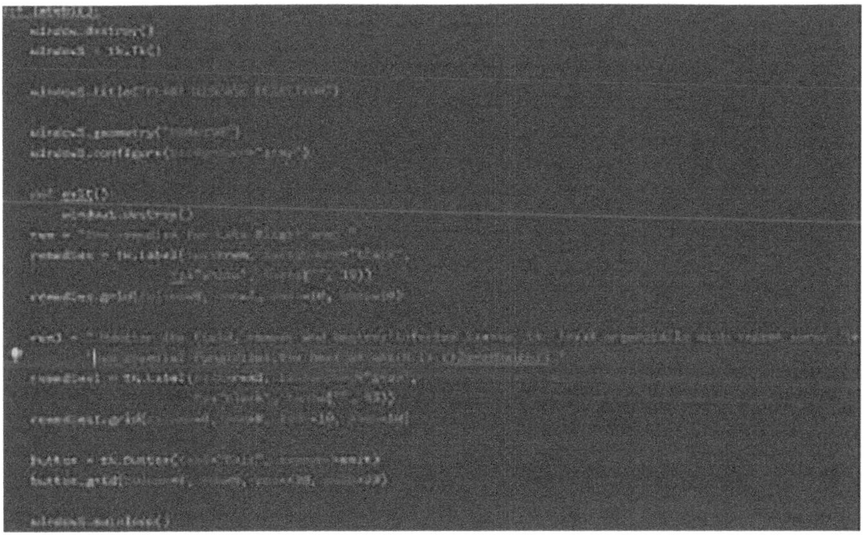

**FIGURE 9.20** Code snippet for creating the window for Late Blight Disease.

```python
if np.argmax(model_out) == 0:
    str_label = 'healthy'
elif np.argmax(model_out) == 1:
    str_label = 'bacterial'
elif np.argmax(model_out) == 2:
    str_label = 'viral'
elif np.argmax(model_out) == 3:
    str_label = 'lateblight'

if str_label =='healthy':
    status ="HEALTHY"
    message = tk.Label(text='Status: ' + status, background="gray",
                       fg="darkgreen", font=("", 15))
else:
    status = "UNHEALTHY"
    message = tk.Label(text='Status: ' + status, background="gray",
                       fg="red", font=("", 15))
```

```python
message.grid(column=0, row=3, padx=10, pady=10)
if str_label == 'bacterial':
    diseasename = "Bacterial Spot "
    disease = tk.Label(text='Disease Name: ' + diseasename, background="gray",
                       fg="red", font=("", 15))
    disease.grid(column=0, row=4, padx=10, pady=10)
    r = tk.Label(text='Click below for remedies...', background="gray", fg="black", font=("", 1
    r.grid(column=0, row=5, padx=10, pady=10)
    button3 = tk.Button(text="Remedies", command=bact)
    button3.grid(column=0, row=6, padx=10, pady=10)
elif str_label == 'viral':
    diseasename = "Yellow leaf curl virus "
    disease = tk.Label(text='Disease Name: ' + diseasename, background="gray",
                       fg="red", font=("", 15))
    disease.grid(column=0, row=4, padx=10, pady=10)
    r = tk.Label(text='Click below for remedies...', background="gray", fg="black", font=("", 1
    r.grid(column=0, row=5, padx=10, pady=10)
    button3 = tk.Button(text="Remedies", command=vir)
```

FIGURE 9.21 Code snippet for determining the class of the test image (pt. 1).

Healthy
Unhealthy
Bacterial Spot
Leaf Curl Virus
Late Blight

Figure 9.23 shows the underlying code snippet to create a window that opens an image to be used as a test image.

```python
elif str_label == 'lateblight':
    diseasename = "Late Blight "
    disease = tk.Label(text='Disease Name: ' + diseasename, background="gray",
                       fg="red", font=("", 15))
    disease.grid(column=0, row=4, padx=10, pady=10)
    r = tk.Label(text='Click below for remedies...', background="gray", fg="black", font=("", 15))
    r.grid(column=0, row=5, padx=10, pady=10)
    button3 = tk.Button(text="Remedies", command=latebl)
    button3.grid(column=0, row=6, padx=10, pady=10)
else:
    r = tk.Label(text='Plant is healthy', background="lightgreen", fg="darkgreen",
                 font=("", 15))
    r.grid(column=0, row=4, padx=10, pady=10)
    button = tk.Button(text="Exit", command=exit)
    button.grid(column=0, row=9, padx=20, pady=20)
```

**FIGURE 9.22** Code snippet for determining the class of the test image (pt. 2).

```python
def openphoto():
    dirPath = "testpicture"
    fileList = os.listdir(dirPath)
    for fileName in fileList:
        os.remove(dirPath + "/" + fileName)

    fileName = askopenfilename(initialdir='C:/Users/C M ARJUN/Documents/final project testing/test', title='Select image for analysis',
                               filetypes=[('image files', '.jpg')])
    dst = "C:/Users/C M ARJUN/Documents/final project testing/testpicture"
    shutil.copy(fileName, dst)
    load = Image.open(fileName)
    render = ImageTk.PhotoImage(load)
    img = tk.Label(image=render, height="250", width="537")
    img.image = render
    img.place(x=0, y=0)
    img.grid(column=0, row=1, padx=10, pady = 10)
    title.destroy()
    button1.destroy()
    button2 = tk.Button(text="Analyse Image", command=analysis)
    button2.grid(column=0, row=2, padx=10, pady = 10)
button1 = tk.Button(text="Get Photo", command = openphoto)
button1.grid(column=0, row=1, padx=10, pady = 10)

window.mainloop()
```

**FIGURE 9.23** Code snippet for creating the window to open the test image.

## 9.6 RESULT

Consequently, we have successfully achieved the capability to discern whether a plant is in good health or is afflicted by a particular disease through the analysis of its leaf.

In instances where the plant is identified as diseased, the system can further determine the specific nature of the ailment and provide the user with potential remedies to mitigate the development of the disease.

In Figure 9.24, the user interface window exhibits functionality for uploading a photo for disease testing. The plant leaf image is loaded and displayed, and a button to analyze the image is presented in Figure 9.25. Subsequently, the plant leaf image undergoes analysis, and the status, along with any identified disease, is displayed, as depicted in Figure 9.26. Furthermore, a button is available to access information on potential remedies.

We employed an open-source tool called TensorBoard, which offers the necessary visualization and tools for conducting machine learning experiments. TensorBoard comprises a set of web applications tailored for inspecting and comprehending TensorFlow runs and graphs. Importantly, it is designed to operate entirely offline, without the need for internet access. This means it can function on a local machine, behind a corporate firewall, or within a data center.

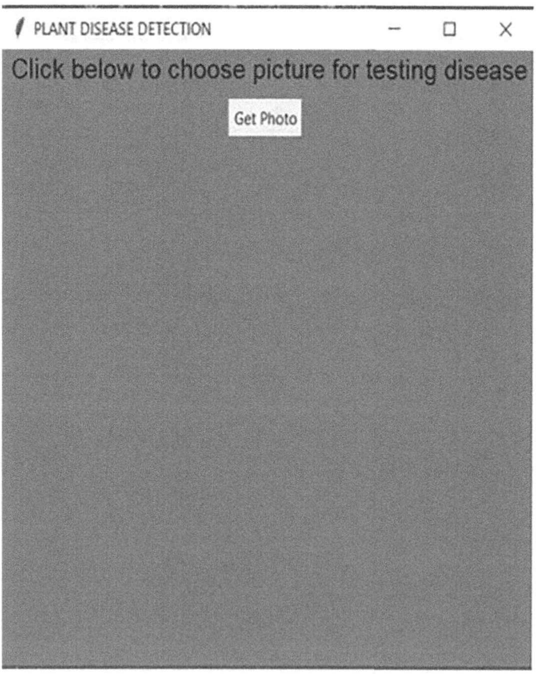


**FIGURE 9.24** UI of the plant disease detection program.

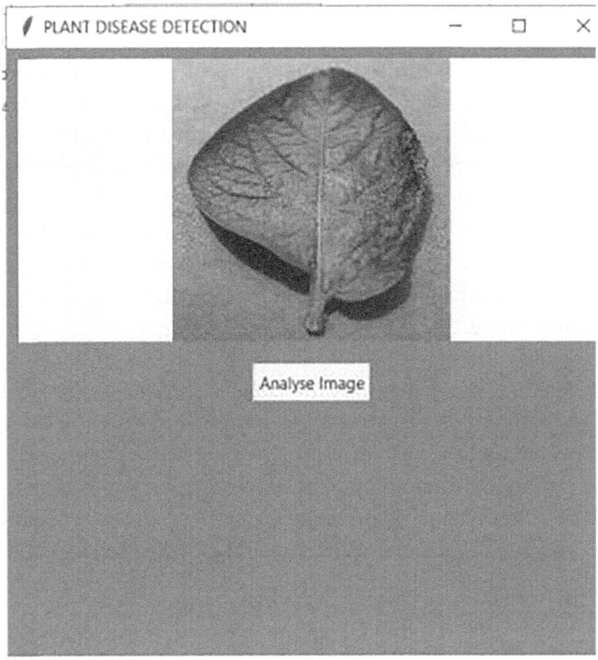


FIGURE 9.25 Uploading the test image onto the UI.

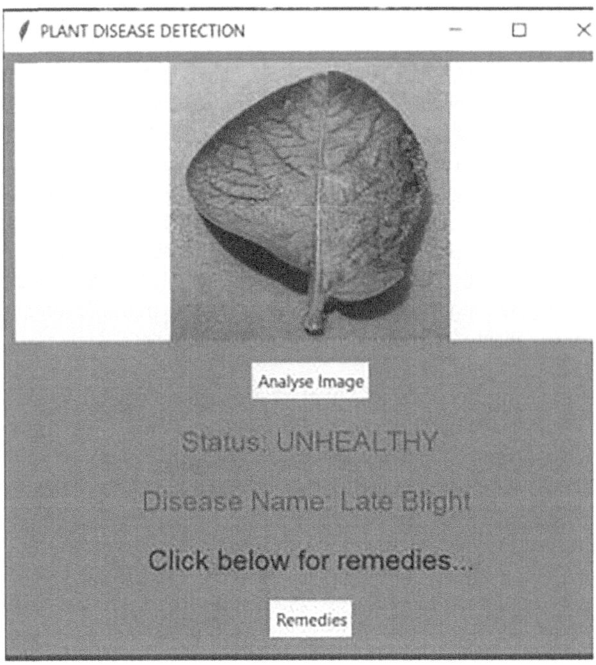


FIGURE 9.26 Status of the test plant leaf image.

## 9.7 CONCLUSION

This chapter presents the achieved outcomes of various disease classification techniques applicable for the detection of plant leaf diseases, along with an algorithm for image segmentation designed for the automatic detection and classification of these diseases. The proposed algorithm was tested on three plant species: tomato, pepper, and potato. Diseases related to these plants were chosen for identification, and the results indicate optimal outcomes with minimal computational efforts. This underscores the efficiency of the proposed algorithm in recognizing and classifying leaf diseases. An added advantage is the system's capability to identify plant diseases at an early or initial stage.

The development of this system was driven by the aim of benefiting farmers and the agricultural sector. The system not only detects diseases in plants but also suggests remedies for combating them. By providing comprehensive knowledge of the disease and appropriate remedies, the system contributes to improving plant health. Operating on Python, the proposed system demonstrates an accuracy rate exceeding 90%.

For future work, the system could be integrated into drones to facilitate aerial surveillance of crop fields. This advancement would enhance the overall monitoring and management of plant health in agricultural settings.

## REFERENCES


1. J. Wen, Y. Shi, X. Zhou, and Y. Xue,"Crop disease classification on inadequate low-resolution target images," *Sensors*, vol. 20, no.16, p. 4601, 2020.
2. M. Atila, M. Uar, K. Akyol, and E. Uar,"Plant leaf disease classification using efficient net deep learning model," *Ecological Informatics,* vol. 61, p. 101182, 2021.
3. T. Wiesner-Hanks, H. Wu, E. Stewart, C. Dechant, and R. J. Nelson, "Millimeter-level plant disease detection from aerial photographs via deep learning and crowd- sourced data," *Frontiers in Plant Science*, vol. 10, p. 1550, 2019.
4. J. G. Barbedo,"Plant disease identification from individual lesions and spots using deep learning," *Biosystems Engineering* , vol. 180, pp.96–107, 2019.
5. Y. Ampatzidis, L. De Bellis, and A. Luvisi, "I Pathology: Robotic applications and management of plants and plant diseases," *Sustainability*, vol. 9, no. 6, p. 1010,2017.
6. A. Breuker's, D. L. Kettenis, M. Mourits, W. V. D. Werf, and A. O. Lansink, "Individual-based models in the analysis of disease transmission in plant production chains: An application to potato brown rot," *Academy of Sciences*, vol. 90, no. 1–3, pp. 112–131,2006.
7. S. Ghosal, D. Blystone, A. K. Singh, B. Ganapathy Subramanian, A. Singh, and S. Sarkar, "An explainable deep machine vision framework for plant stress phenotyping," *Proceedings of the National Academy of Sciences*, vol. 115, no. 18, pp. 4613–4618,2018.
8. E.-C. Oerke, "Crop losses to pests," *Journal of Agricultural Science*, vol. 144, no. 1, pp. 31–43, 2006.
9. X. E. Pantazi, D. Moshou, and A. A. Tamouridou, "Automated leaf disease detection in different crop species through image features analysis and One Class Classifiers," *Computers and Electronics in Agriculture*, vol. 156, pp. 96–104, 2019.
10. J. G. A. Barbedo, "Factors influencing the use of deep learning for plant disease recognition," *Biosystems Engineering*, vol. 172, pp. 84–91,2018.

11. G. Geetha Ramani and J. Arun Pandian, "Identification of plant leaf diseases using a nine-layer deep convolutional neural network," *Computers & Electrical Engineering*, vol. 76, pp. 323–338, 2019.
12. P. F. Konstantinos, "Deep learning models for plant disease detection and diagnosis," *Computers & Electrical Engineering*, vol. 145, pp. 311–318,2018.

# Index